THE ESSEN~~TIAL GUIDE~~
DOING ~~A~~
SOCIAL CAI~~RE LITERATURE~~

~~REVIEW~~

This step-by-step guide takes the reader logically through the process of undertaking a literature review, from determining when this methodology might be useful, through to publishing the findings. It is designed particularly for students undertaking a dissertation using literature review methodology. However, it also caters for practitioners who wish to review the existing evidence in order to develop practice.

Key features of the text include:

- a chapter on what makes a good literature review, so that readers are clear and confident about what they're aiming for;
- discussion of the value of literature reviews, whether for fulfilling the requirements of a course or for developing practice;
- a chapter structure that reflects the structure of a typical dissertation by literature review, making the material intuitive and easy to navigate;
- case examples throughout to illustrate how methodological principles work in practice;
- a troubleshooting guide to provide support and advice on common problems when carrying out a literature review;
- advice on the dissemination of findings.

Written by an established author with significant experience teaching and supervising students doing literature reviews, this invaluable text offers systematic and insightful advice on all aspects of literature review methodology, from problem identification to synthesizing information to forming conclusions. It is ideal for any student or practitioner in health and social care looking to undertake a literature review for study or practice purposes.

Jaqui Hewitt-Taylor is a Senior Lecturer in Practice Development at the Faculty of Health and Social Sciences at Bournemouth University, UK. She has a wealth of experience teaching in research and offering support as a tutor and supervisor for dissertations at undergraduate and postgraduate levels. Her most recent books are *Developing Person-Centred Practice* (2015) and *Managing Change in Healthcare: A Step by Step Guide* (2013).

THE ESSENTIAL GUIDE TO DOING A HEALTH AND SOCIAL CARE LITERATURE REVIEW

Jaqui Hewitt-Taylor

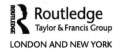

Routledge
Taylor & Francis Group

LONDON AND NEW YORK

First published 2017
by Routledge
2 Park Square, Milton Park, Abingdon, Oxon OX14 4RN

and by Routledge
711 Third Avenue, New York, NY 10017

Routledge is an imprint of the Taylor & Francis Group, an informa business

British Library Cataloguing-in-Publication Data
A catalogue record for this book is available from the British Library

Library of Congress Cataloging in Publication Data
Names: Hewitt-Taylor, Jaqui, author.
Title: The essential guide to doing a health and social care literature
review / Jaqui Hewitt-Taylor.
Description: Abingdon, Oxon ; New York, NY : Routledge, 2017.
Identifiers: LCCN 2016046383 | ISBN 9781138186910 (hardback)
| ISBN 9781138186927 (pbk.) | ISBN 9781315643472 (ebook)
Subjects: | MESH: Health Services Research–methods | Review
Literature as Topic | Abstracting and Indexing as Topic | Research
Design
Classification: LCC RA409 | NLM W 84.3 | DDC
362.1072/3–dc23
LC record available at https://lccn.loc.gov/2016046383

ISBN: 978-1-138-18691-0 (hbk)
ISBN: 978-1-138-18692-7 (pbk)
ISBN: 978-1-315-64347-2 (ebk)

Typeset in Goudy
by Wearset Ltd, Boldon, Tyne and Wear

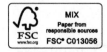

MIX
Paper from
responsible sources
FSC
www.fsc.org   FSC® C013056

Printed and bound in Great Britain by
TJ International Ltd, Padstow, Cornwall

Contents

Illustrations

Figures

Tables

Acknowledgements

I acknowledge with thanks my eleven-year-old son John's assistance with the writing of this book: providing me with much needed breaks to play with Lego, trains, and to try to master the art of Minecraft.

Chapter 1
What is literature review methodology?

It is generally agreed that practice should be based on the current best evidence. However, in order to achieve this, we need to know what the current best evidence is. Literature review methodology can be a useful part of establishing this.

Not all the evidence that exists is good evidence, so it is necessary to evaluate any evidence that we find, or are presented with, in order to determine how much heed should be paid to it. In addition, there is often more than one piece of evidence on a given subject, and the actions recommended across sources are not always consistent. Finally, some evidence is perfectly good for what it claims to be, but is not sufficient, of itself, to really convince us that it should be acted on. Therefore, in order for our practice to be directed by the current best evidence, all the existing information on a subject needs to be identified, evaluated and synthesized so that the nature and strength of that evidence when viewed as a whole is known.

Despite the desirability of identifying the current composite best evidence in this way, the ever-increasing body of literature related to health and social care can make it very difficult for individual practitioners to achieve in any field of practice (Uman 2011). Good quality reviews of the existing literature, that provide a rigorously derived summary of what is and is not currently known about a subject, and the strength of the evidence that exists, can therefore be very useful. Nonetheless, like any evidence, in order to be useful, such reviews must themselves be of good quality. One intention of this book is to explore, step by step, the process of using literature review methodology to conduct a rigorous review of the existing literature on a particular subject. First, though, what a study that uses literature review methodology is requires clarification.

1.1 What is a literature review?

A literature review is exactly what the name suggests: a review of the existing literature on a subject. However, the term encompasses a number of different types of review, ranging from essays that do not claim to be particularly rigorous or systematic, through to systematic reviews (Aveyard 2014: 2–3). All of these approaches gather and present existing literature on a particular subject. However, the level of rigour with which reviews are conducted, and whether their intention is to identify, analyse and collate all the existing literature on a specific topic, varies, depending upon the type of review in question.

At the top end of the quality scale of reviews of the literature in terms of rigour and system are systematic reviews, such as those published by the Cochrane Collaboration. These are high-quality reviews of all the available evidence on a subject (Aveyard 2014: 2–3). They systematically and exhaustively search for and evaluate all the available evidence on the subject in question, including the unpublished literature, and articles that are not in the reviewers' first languages. The studies for inclusion in the review are selected using predefined eligibility criteria, and the review is conducted using a clearly stated and reproducible methodology (Higgins and Green 2011). This type of review is generally undertaken by a team of researchers and requires considerable time and resources (Aveyard 2014: 2–3). At the other end of the spectrum in terms of the required level of rigour and system are documents that are described as literature reviews, but are really essays in which some of the literature on a subject is presented. Such reviews do not claim to follow a rigorous or systematic process, or to include all the literature related to the subject in question.

Studies that use literature review methodology fall somewhere between the two types of review described above. They aim to critically evaluate the existing evidence on a subject and to develop a narrative that presents the composite best evidence concerning this (Roberts and Bailey 2010). However, they are not required to be as exhaustive as a systematic review (for example, there is generally no expectation that literature in languages that the reviewer does not speak will be accessed and translated). This is in part because studies that use literature review methodology do not necessarily have a team of researchers involved: often, they are the work of a sole person, with limited funding. There are many situations in which this type of review can be very valuable. For instance, an individual or small team may want to evaluate and collate the existing evidence about something relevant to their day-to-day practice, but may not have the time or resources to conduct a full systematic review. In such situations, literature review methodology can be used to carry out a smaller scale, less exhaustive, but still systematic and rigorous, review of the current evidence regarding a particular issue (Cronin *et al.* 2008; Roberts and Bailey 2010; Aveyard 2014: 2–3).

1.2 Literature review methodology as secondary research

Because it is designed to be a rigorous and systematic form of enquiry, literature review methodology can be described as a form of secondary research. The distinction between primary and secondary research is that in primary research original data are collected and analysed (Aveyard 2014). In contrast, in secondary research, data that have already been collected and analysed are gathered, in order to explore what the existing evidence shows when seen as a composite whole. In effect, literature review methodology therefore uses existing literature as its data. However, to earn the title of secondary research, a literature review must meet the quality standards of research: it must follow a process that is systematic, rigorous, and minimizes the risk of the apparent findings being due to chance, errors or bias (Cronin *et al.* 2008, Aveyard 2014: 3–4). In order to achieve this, several discrete steps should be followed when carrying out a study using literature review methodology, as shown in Box 1.1. Each stage is equally

---

Box 1.1

Steps required in a study that uses literature review methodology

- Identify the need for a review.
- Determine the focus of the review.
- Devise the review question, aims and objectives.
- Develop the search strategy.
- Formulate clear inclusion and exclusion criteria.
- Carry out the search.
- Record details of the search, the documents retrieved and the decisions made about their inclusion or exclusion from the review.
- Appraise each individual piece of evidence.
- Synthesize the findings from across all the evidence.
- Draw conclusions.
- Make recommendations.
- Consider ways in which to disseminate the findings from the review.

important in ensuring that the process as a whole is rigorous and systematic. The rest of this book describes and discusses these stages of the literature review process.

1.3 Overview of the book

The remainder of this book is divided into two parts: the first explores the context and background of literature review methodology: some of the reasons why a literature review might be conducted, and the characteristics of a good review. The second part deals with the process and practicalities of conducting a study that uses literature review methodology.

In the first part of the book, Chapter 2 discusses some of the circumstances in which conducting a literature review can be useful, including both practice-based and academic situations. The chapter is divided into three main sections: first, carrying out a literature review to fulfil some of the requirements of a programme of study; second, carrying out a literature review because of a problem that has been identified in practice and, finally, carrying out a literature review to support and further develop an area of good practice.

Having identified in Chapter 2 some of the circumstances in which using literature review methodology might be useful, Chapter 3 provides an overview of what constitutes a good quality review of the literature. This chapter focuses on the need for the study as a whole to be systematic, rigorous, unbiased, and for the rationales for the decisions made to be explicit. However, it also highlights the purpose and importance of each of the key stages within a study that uses literature review methodology. These stages then form the individual chapters of the second part of the book.

In the second section of this book, the individual methodological steps required to conduct a good quality review of the literature are discussed, with one chapter devoted to each step.

Chapter 4 addresses the background to, and rationale for, carrying out a review of the literature. It outlines how the documentation of the background reading that informs the development of the review question differs from the in-depth evaluation of the existing evidence that constitutes the main body of the review. It also discusses the type of information that might be incorporated in the background and rationale sections of a review, and how they can be structured so as to lead logically to the review's question and aims.

Chapter 5 focuses on the development of the review's question, aims and objectives. It discusses the importance of having a clear, focused and answerable question, how this can be achieved, and the consequences of it not being accomplished. It then explores the development of aims that will enable the review question to be answered, and that are realistic and achievable. The chapter goes on to differentiate the aims of the review from its objectives, describing the value of having specific objectives, but the need for these to be congruent with the study question and aims.

Chapter 6 outlines the process of conducting a search for evidence that will address the review's question and aims, including the development of a search strategy, and the practicalities of carrying out a search. It discusses ways of breaking the study question into key concepts, including the use of tools such as PICO, SPICE and *SPIDER* to achieve this. It then goes on to describe the process of identifying keywords and their synonyms, using Boolean operators, truncation and wildcards, and the importance of having clear inclusion and exclusion criteria for the review. This is followed by an exploration of the decisions that need to be made regarding how to source literature, and the types of literature that will be included in the review. Finally, the practicalities of conducting the search, recording the results of the search, and steps that can be taken if the initial search yields inadequate or excessive numbers of papers are discussed.

Chapter 7 explores the next stage in the literature review process: appraising the literature that has been gathered for review. It begins with an explanation of the importance of this step being systematically and rigorously undertaken, and the value of using specifically designed tools to assist in achieving this. The chapter then discusses the general principles of appraising research, before entering into an exploration of the particulars of appraising qualitative, quantitative and mixed methods research. The chapter ends by discussing how other forms of evidence such as evaluation, audit, expert opinion and case reports can be appraised.

Chapter 8 moves on from the process of appraising each individual piece of evidence included in the review to a discussion of the process of synthesizing the evidence from across sources. It begins with an overview of some of the approaches that can be used for the synthesis of qualitative, quantitative and mixed methods studies, such as meta-analysis and meta-synthesis. However, these types of synthesis are often not appropriate for a study that uses literature review methodology. Therefore, the main focus of the chapter is on narrative approaches to the synthesis of evidence from sources that are heterogeneous, and potentially include both research and non-research evidence.

Chapter 9 takes the process of literature review methodology to the stage beyond the findings from the review, to the discussion of these findings. It outlines the purpose of the discussion section of a study that uses literature review methodology, and explores what should be included in it. It also highlights how the discussion of the findings from the review should enable these to be distinguished from, but also located within, the existing body of evidence on the subject in question.

Chapter 10 explores the final element of a study that uses literature review methodology: the drawing of conclusions and making of recommendations. It outlines the need to ensure that the conclusions are derived from the findings, that they are clearly stated, answer the initial study question, and address its aims. The chapter then discusses the making of recommendations from the literature review's findings, emphasizing the need for there to be a clear relationship between the study question, aims, findings, conclusions and recommendations.

Chapter 11 goes beyond the final stage of conducting a study that uses literature review methodology, by discussing approaches to disseminating the findings from the review. In this chapter, the value of sharing the findings from a review of the literature is outlined, followed by ways in which this may be achieved, including publication, conference presentations and electronic media.

The final chapter of the book summarizes the key points from the preceding chapters, and re-emphasizes the need for literature review methodology to use systemic, rigorous and unbiased processes. The book itself concludes with a troubleshooting guide that addresses problems that are commonly encountered in carrying out a literature review. It discusses each of these briefly, but also refers back to key chapters where fuller information on each issue can be found.

Part 1

The context and background of literature review methodology

Chapter 2
Why carry out a review of the literature?

Key points:

- Literature review methodology enables information from across sources to be identified, analysed and synthesized. This approach can therefore be very useful for clarifying what the current best evidence about a particular subject is.
- Using literature review methodology is often an option for fulfilling the dissertation requirements of a programme of academic study.
- Literature review methodology can be a useful part of resolving a problem in practice, as it enables the composite evidence concerning potential solutions to be established. However, before undertaking a review of the literature, it is important to ensure that the problem, and its possible causes, has been accurately identified.
- Literature review methodology may assist in sustaining and developing good practice by providing evidence about how positive aspects of current practice can be further advanced.

Literature review methodology can be useful in a number of circumstances. There are times when there seem to be many different views on the right, or best, way to approach a situation, all accompanied by evidence of one sort or another, but a lack of clarity concerning what is actually the best thing to do. Carrying out a literature review in such situations can enable you to gather all the available evidence on the subject in question, ascertain exactly what each piece of evidence says, evaluate its quality, and thus determine what the composite best evidence is. Using literature review methodology can also be advantageous when a number of pieces of information about an aspect of practice exist, but where none of these, individually, presents sufficiently strong or conclusive evidence to merit action. There may, for instance, be a number of small studies, opinion papers or case reports, about an aspect of practice. All of these may be perfectly good for the type of evidence that they claim to be, but none may, of themselves, make you feel really confident about following their suggestions. In such a situation, gathering all the available information together, evaluating it, and determining the overall evidence from across sources, can enable you to decide whether or not the collective strength of the existing evidence merits action. This can be useful for informing practice, and determining whether further research is needed (and if so what direction that research should take). Using literature review methodology can therefore be very useful for the purpose of answering questions that ask: 'What is the evidence for...', 'What evidence exists about...' or 'What is the strength of the evidence concerning...'.

Although questions of this type are particularly amenable to the use of literature review methodology, a variety of situations or events can be the catalyst that leads you to ask: 'Would it be useful to conduct a literature review about this?'. These include: undertaking a programme of study that includes the requirement to carry out a dissertation; identifying an issue that has become problematic in practice and wanting to explore the evidence concerning possible solutions; and seeking to build upon and further develop good practice. These three situations are often linked: for instance, if you are undertaking a dissertation as part of an academic programme it makes sense to use this as an opportunity to explore something that will be useful to you in practice. Therefore, although these three situations are described separately in the rest of this chapter, in reality, they frequently overlap with one another.

2.1 Using literature review methodology to fulfil part of a course of academic study

Using literature review methodology is often an option for fulfilling the dissertation element of a programme of academic study. Making the right decision about whether or not to use literature review as the methodology for your dissertation before embarking on it is important because if not time can be wasted on beginning to undertake what will become an unsuccessful study. In addition, knowing that you have chosen an appropriate methodological approach for your dissertation should enable you to feel convinced that your study will make a meaningful contribution to the existing body of knowledge. This may be important in assisting you to maintain your motivation whilst you work on your dissertation.

When you are planning your dissertation, you may feel that conducting a literature review will not produce as much new or valuable knowledge as carrying out a piece of primary research, because the evidence that you are collating already exists. As Chapter 1 identified, literature review methodology is a form of secondary research, and this term can imply that it is in some way the second-class option compared to primary research. However, if used for the right thing, and conducted systematically and rigorously, a literature review can be as, and even more, valuable as primary research. It depends on what information is needed to answer the question that you have, and what evidence already exists about the subject in question. There may already be plenty of evidence (in the form of research, expert opinion or case reports) about a particular subject, but no review that draws all this information together. In such a situation, conducting a literature review to evaluate and collate the existing evidence would probably be more useful than carrying out another fairly small piece of primary research. Alternatively, if there is very little, or no, existing evidence on a subject, primary research would be the better option for your dissertation. Box 2.1 shows a case study of how someone might select an appropriate methodology for their dissertation.

Box 2.1

Choosing an appropriate approach for a dissertation

Edward is a public health practitioner who is currently undertaking his MSc degree. He is particularly interested in reducing teenage substance misuse. For the dissertation element of his programme of study he had, therefore, initially planned to carry out a piece of primary research exploring practitioners' experiences of different approaches to reducing substance misuse amongst teenagers. However, on reading around the subject, he found that there was already a lot of evidence available on this topic, but that it was of variable quality, provided inconsistent advice, and thus did not give a clear overall indication of what works best. This made him wonder if it would be more useful to spend his time systematically and rigorously gathering the existing evidence on this subject, evaluating and synthesizing it. This seemed likely to enable him to gain a clearer view of what was already known about the subject, in order to provide direction for practice. It would also highlight any gaps in existing knowledge, which would be useful for informing future research.

Do not assume that a particular methodological approach is, in principle, the best for your dissertation. The best approach will depend on what you want to explore, and what your study question is.

When you are deciding whether or not to use literature review methodology for your dissertation it is therefore important to have a good idea of what evidence already exists on the subject in question, and whether this has already been collated (for example in a literature review or systematic review). This enables you to decide whether or not literature review methodology would be an appropriate approach to adopt. For instance, if you work on a neonatal intensive care unit, you might decide that you want to focus your dissertation on parents' experiences of their newborn baby being critically ill. An initial search of the literature might reveal that a number of studies have already been carried out in this area, but that there is no existing review that collates all this evidence. Such a discovery might lead you to decide that carrying out a study using literature review methodology would be a valuable contribution to knowledge in this field. This would enable you to clarify what is known, but also what is not known, about the subject, and would be useful for your own practice. In addition, it would make a valuable contribution to the knowledge available within the neonatal intensive care community.

Another reason to select to use literature review methodology for your dissertation is that the skills it requires are a useful acquisition for future situations where you may want to ascertain the evidence about something. This might include finding out the best way to approach a particular aspect of your day-to-day practice, or to assist you in developing guidelines, protocols or policies that need to be based on the current best evidence. Developing the skills required to systematically and rigorously appraise and collate the current evidence on a particular subject will also be useful for any further academic study that you undertake. The prime reason for selecting a particular methodology for your dissertation should always be that it matches the subject that you want to investigate. Nonetheless, if you have an interest in this methodology, or want to develop and hone your skills in critically evaluating and synthesizing evidence, it can be a useful choice to make, provided it is compatible with the subject that you plan to investigate.

Finally, when undertaking a course of academic study, pragmatic considerations often come into play. Depending on your time and other commitments, it may be more practical to undertake a literature review than a piece of primary research. This does not mean that it is an easier option. In some respects it can be more challenging, and requires equally in-depth and robust knowledge of research methodology, and rigour and system in conducting the study as primary research does. However, the practical challenges it presents are different. A study that uses literature review methodology seldom requires the approval of an ethics committee, as no new data is collected, which can be useful when time is short. In addition, although obtaining and evaluating literature from various sources requires considerable time, this time tends to be able to be organized slightly more flexibly than that which is required for conducting primary research. For example, literature can be searched for at any hour of the day and can often be searched for from home. These considerations should never be the overwhelming reason for using literature review methodology for your dissertation. They can, however, be added to the melting pot of decision-making when you are considering how to make your dissertation achievable, but also relevant to your practice, and of good quality.

There are, nonetheless, times when using literature review methodology will not be a good choice for your dissertation. The most obvious is when there is not enough literature on the subject for you to be able to carry out a review. Whilst, as Chapter 7 discusses, all of the evidence that you use in a literature review need not be derived from research, there does have to be enough literature for your dissertation to be of sufficient quality and depth. If there is not very much evidence already available concerning the subject that you have chosen, it probably indicates that a study that uses primary research, rather than literature review methodology, is needed.

When you select the subject and methodology that you will use to fulfil the dissertation requirements of a programme of study, the reasons for your choices will often be linked to your practice. This might be because you want to address a problem that has arisen in practice, or because you have identified an area of good practice and want to develop it further.

Pitfall to avoid

It can be tempting to think that using literature review methodology is the least demanding choice for a dissertation. However, it requires as much time, effort and knowledge as primary research.

2.2 Using literature review methodology to assist in resolving a problem in practice

When a problem has been identified in practice, literature review methodology can be a useful part of the process of determining the best way to address the problem, or of finding a better or more effective way to work. However, if a literature review is being carried out in response to a problem in practice, an important precursor to performing the review is to be clear about exactly what the problem that needs to be addressed is. Otherwise, there is a risk that your review question and aims, however diligently developed, will not address the core of the problem that you are seeking to resolve.

> **Pitfall to avoid**
>
> Avoid seeking the solution to a problem before being really sure of what the problem is.

2.2.1 Problem identification

Before seeking a solution to what appears to be a problem it is first expedient to consider what evidence there is to support there actually being a problem. For example, the introduction of electronic prescribing on a ward might appear to have been followed by an increase in the number of medication errors made. Before considering what actions should be taken to address the problem it would, however, be worthwhile to check whether more errors had really been made since the introduction of the new system. It might, in fact, be that the new system enabled more robust and accurate error reporting than was possible previously. Distinguishing whether an apparent rise in the number of errors made in the administration of medications represented more errors being made, or more errors being detected, would therefore be important. Otherwise, in an attempt to address the problem that appeared to exist, a change might be made that simply returned the ward to a system that was less robust at detecting errors.

If it becomes clear that a problem does indeed exist, the next stage in the process of problem identification is to ascertain whether what appears to be the difficulty is really what is problematic (Garavaglia 2008; Okes 2008). It is quite common for what initially seems to be the problem to really be either the effect of the problem, or something that is in fact nothing to do with the problem (Randall 2011). Before beginning to develop a literature review question in response to a problem in practice it is therefore always worth taking some time to ensure that you know, as precisely as possible, what the problem is. Otherwise, even if all the available evidence is diligently sought, evaluated, collated and acted on, the presenting problem is likely to remain unresolved because it has not really been addressed (Randall 2011). The only thing that will have been achieved is that time and resources will have been expended on finding, and possibly trying to implement, a solution to the wrong problem, or to the effects of a problem rather than its cause (Parkin 2009: 147–9).

If, for instance, the introduction of electronic prescribing on a particular ward has been followed by an increase in the number of medication errors, the assumption might be that the new system of prescribing is the cause. As a result, a review of the literature concerning the safety of electronic prescribing might appear to be in order, so as to identify solutions to the problem of this approach causing errors in the administration of medication. Such a review might reveal a number of possible solutions, including additional training, revising the way that prescriptions are carried out, or making more computers available. However, the problem might in fact be that the ward was unusually short-staffed at the time when electronic prescribing was introduced, and was using a lot of temporary staff who were unfamiliar with the most commonly used medications. If this were the real reason for the increase in medication errors, then taking steps to address problems with electronic prescribing per se, even if based on the current best evidence, would not resolve the problem. These actions might even divert resources that could have been used to improve staffing into areas that were not actually causing any problems (such as purchasing additional computer hardware). Identifying what the problem that requires addressing really is therefore forms a vital stage of using literature review methodology as a part of addressing a problem in practice.

When you are seeking to solve a problem it is, then, important to look beyond the superficial, and challenge immediate assumptions about what the problem is. A part of this may involve looking at when, where and in what circumstances the apparent problem has occurred, to see if this provides any information about its possible cause or causes (Okes 2008). In the example of there appearing to be an increase in medication errors following the introduction of electronic prescribing, this might include checking: staffing levels when the problem became apparent compared to what they were previously; the skill mix on the ward at the time when the problem occurred compared to previous times; what medication the errors were made with; when the errors were made and who made them. This type of information could confirm your initial thoughts about what the problem is, but might equally introduce new ideas about potential causes. It does not necessarily show the root cause of the problem, but it may give useful initial information about directions to follow in seeking its cause or causes.

Although any problem in practice matters, most workplaces have a number of competing demands on their time and resources, and, even if a problem does exist, a decision has to be made about the priority that it should be afforded. Noting how often a problem occurs, as well as where and when it happens, helps to gauge how serious, or urgent, addressing it is (Okes 2008).

Ascertaining the type of information described above would give a good indication of whether an apparent problem really exists, what it is, its scale, and the degree of urgency with which it needs to be addressed. Identifying in these general terms what the problem is, and whether it merits attention, may be all that is needed for you to begin to find a solution. For example, if it has been shown that the move to electronic prescribing is in fact the problem, a literature review that asks the question: 'What is the safest way to approach electronic prescribing?' might be appropriate. However, sometimes identifying the problem is not enough, and the root cause of that problem needs to be sought before an effective solution can be devised. Otherwise, there is still a risk that the effects of the problem, not its cause, will be addressed (Okes 2008).

If, for instance, a decrease in staffing levels rather than electronic prescribing was shown to be the cause of an increase in medication errors, the logical solution might appear to be to employ more staff. However, it would still be useful to look a little deeper into why there were poor staffing levels at the time in case there was a particular problem that caused staff to be dissatisfied and leave the ward. If not, new staff might be recruited, only to leave because the problem that caused staff dissatisfaction remained unresolved. To achieve this deeper analysis of the situation in question, problem analysis processes may be useful.

2.2.2 Problem analysis processes

Establishing how or why various elements of a situation contribute to any problem that has been identified is an important part of developing effective solutions. A problem is also often the result of more than one cause. Identifying whether a variety of causes have united to create one problem, whether all of them can be addressed, and if not which should be the priority are therefore useful steps in the process of addressing problems in practice.

When you are looking at problems in your own workplace, it can be hard to completely put aside your assumptions and personal opinions about the situation (Paton and McCalman 2008: 240). For example, you might know that several members of staff on your ward felt unhappy about moving to electronic prescribing because of a lack of computer hardware. You might also be aware that, since the introduction of electronic prescribing, people have been complaining about the lack of computers available to access prescriptions. It would therefore be easy to think that as you know this lack of resources to be problematic, you can safely assume that it is the main cause of any increase in medication errors since the introduction of electronic prescribing. However, this may not be the cause, or the only cause, of the problem, and seeking a solution based on this assumption might, consequently, not lead to a lasting improvement. It can, therefore, sometimes be useful to use a problem analysis process which encourages you to gain as objective a view of the situation as possible, and to think deeply and widely about all the possible causes of any problem that you are unpicking.

Various problem analysis tools exist, each of which have particular pros and cons. One that is commonly used is known as the Five Whys approach: a tool that was originally developed in order to identify the root causes of problems in the manufacturing and production industries (Kohfeldt and Langhaut 2011). The Five Whys approach seeks to establish the cause or causes of a problem by changing a statement of a problem into a question that asks why, and then asking more 'why' questions about it until the root cause of the problem is ascertained (Latino 2004; Kohfeldt and Langhaut 2011). In the case of an increased number of medication errors being reported following the introduction of electronic prescribing, the initial problem statement might be: 'There has been an increase in the number of medication errors reported in the past two months'. (Electronic prescribing, despite being assumed to be a part of the problem, is removed from the problem statement, as it has not yet been confirmed as a cause.) The why question developed from this problem statement could be: 'Why has there been an increase in the number of medication errors reported in the last two months?' The answers to that 'why' question might include: 'Because people are not sufficiently familiar with the new electronic prescribing process', 'Because there are not enough computer resources so people feel rushed when checking and administering drugs', and 'Because staffing levels have fallen in the past two months'. These answers to the initial question are followed by repeatedly asking 'why' about each answer until the root cause or causes of the problem become clear. These causes can then be used as a basis for considering possible solutions to the problem.

Although this approach is known as the Five Whys, the number five is an approximate value: the principle is that it is necessary to continue to ask 'why' until no further why questions would be helpful (Latino 2004; Randall 2011). How the whys are recorded depends on individual preference, but they are often presented as a table or a Fishbone Diagram, as shown in Table 2.1 and Figure 2.1. Alongside the answer to each 'why' it is useful to note the source of evidence that informs the response, so that the certainty with which this is known can be gauged (Latino 2004). As shown in Table 2.1, this approach might enable the cause of the problem to move beyond being seen as a combination of staffing issues, inadequate computer hardware, and unfamiliarity with the process of electronic prescribing. It could demonstrate that whilst the superficiality of the training package used is problematic, the lack of resources to enable staff to seek to move beyond the superficial in completing the training package augments this problem. In this instance, in order to be effective, any solution to the problem would need to address both these issues.

Another approach to problem analysis is to use what is known as the Fishbone Diagram. This approach documents problems and their possible causes by depicting them as a fish skeleton: the head of the fish represents the problem and the contributory factors are shown as the spines (Iles and Cranfield 2004; Yazdani and Tavakkoli-Moghaddam 2012). When a Fishbone Diagram is used as a way of documenting a Five Whys analysis, the head is used to present the initial 'why' question. The spines then represent the answers to the first 'why' question, with smaller bones added to the spines to explore these answers in more detail. If a Fishbone Diagram was used to document the Five Whys analysis concerning errors in medication administration following the introduction of electronic prescribing, it might look something like that shown in Figure 2.1.

A third way of analysing the cause (or causes) of a problem is to use the process of Problem Tree analysis (also referred to as Situational Analysis). This approach uses the image of a tree to structure and illustrate the exploration of a problem. Like the Five Whys analysis and Fishbone Diagram, Problem Tree analysis aims to distinguish the causes and the effects of a problem, so as to ensure that any solutions devised address the former rather than the latter (Hovland 2005). The process begins with a starter problem being documented (for example, an increase in the number of medication errors). From this, related problems or issues are identified. The causes of the

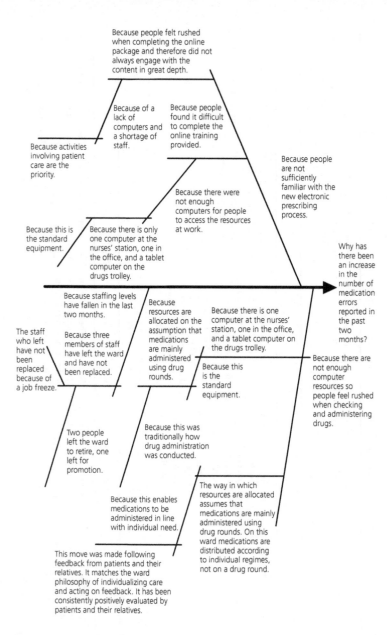

Figure 2.1 The Fishbone Diagram: why has there been an increase in the number of medication errors reported in the past two months?

Table 2.1 The Five Whys: why has there been an increase in the number of medication errors reported in the past two months?

Because people are not sufficiently familiar with the new electronic prescribing process. (Evidence: discussions with staff)	Because there are not enough computer resources so people feel rushed when checking and administering drugs. (Evidence: discussions with staff)		Because staffing levels have fallen in the last two months. (Evidence: discussions with staff and examining staff rotas)
Why?	*Why?*		*Why?*
Because the online training provided was difficult for people to complete. (Evidence: discussions with staff)	Because there is only one computer at the nurses' station, one in the office, and a tablet computer on the drugs trolley. (Evidence: discussions with staff and observation of ward equipment)	The way in which resources are allocated assumes that medications are mainly administered using drug rounds, whereas on this ward medications are distributed according to individual regimes, not on a drug round. (Evidence: discussions with ward staff)	Because three members of staff have left the ward and have not been replaced. (Evidence: discussions with staff and comparing staff rotas over the past six months)
Why?	*Why?*	*Why?*	*Why?*
Because there were not enough computers for people to access the resources at work. (Evidence: discussions with staff, observation of computer usage on the ward)	Because this is the standard equipment. (Evidence: Trust IT policy)	Because the belief is that this enables medications to be administered in line with individual need. (Evidence: discussions with ward staff)	Two people left the ward to retire. One left for promotion. (Evidence: discussion with ward manager)
Because people felt rushed when completing the online package and therefore did not always engage with the content in great depth. (Evidence: discussions with staff)			*Why?*
			The staff who left have not been replaced because of a job freeze. (Evidence: discussion with ward manager)

Why?	Why?	Why?	Why?
Because there is only one computer at the nurses' station, one in the office, and a tablet computer on the drugs trolley. (Evidence: observation of ward equipment)	Because of a lack of computers and shortage of staff. (Evidence: discussions with staff and evidence of staff vacancies on the rota)	Because resource allocation assumes that medications are mainly administered on drug rounds, making one tablet computer located on the drugs trolley adequate for drug administration purposes. (Evidence: discussions with staff and Trust IT services)	This move was made following feedback from patients and their relatives. It matches the ward philosophy of individualizing care and acting on feedback. It has been consistently positively evaluated by patients and their relatives. (Evidence: discussions with ward staff)
Why?	Why?	Why?	
Because this is the standard equipment. (Evidence: Trust IT policy)	Because direct patient care activities take priority. (Evidence: discussions with staff)	Because this is the usual approach to drug administration. (Evidence: discussions with staff and Trust IT department)	

problem are placed at the lower part of the diagram, and become the tree's roots, and those that are the effects or consequences of it are put higher up, and become the branches (European Commission 2004). When an issue is identified, the question: 'What causes this?' is posed, so that cause and effect are distinguished and each statement can be placed appropriately in the overall picture of the problem situation. During the process of exploring the problem, statements may move between being seen as the roots or branches of the tree. However, by the end of the process, the causes should be clearly located as the roots of the tree. It is these that need to be addressed in order to effectively resolve the problem. A Problem Tree diagram exploring the issue of the increased number of medication errors following the introduction of electronic prescribing might be something like that shown in Figure 2.2.

The Seven S model (Iles and Cranfield 2004, Cameron and Green 2009: 122) is a fourth approach to problem analysis. This model maps out the key elements of a team or organization, the roles that they might play in a problem that has been identified, and how these interact with each other. The elements represented by the Seven Ss are:

- strategy;
- structure;
- systems;
- staff;
- style of management;
- shared beliefs/values;
- skills.

(Iles and Cranfield 2004; Cameron and Green 2009: 122)

Using this approach to explore an increase in the number of medication errors following the introduction of electronic prescribing might include thinking about: what staff are needed to prevent medication errors; what skills these staff would need when using electronic prescribing; whether these are currently available; and what systems are in place to ensure that staff gain these skills. Any one of the 'Ss' may fall into more than one category: staff experience or expertise, for instance, might fall within both 'skills' and 'staffing'. It is also useful to map the Ss against each other to see how one may influence the rest, so as to gain a complete picture of the potentially interlinking causes of problem situations. A ward might, for example, have encountered difficulty with using electronic prescribing because there were not enough computer resources available (a problem with 'structure').

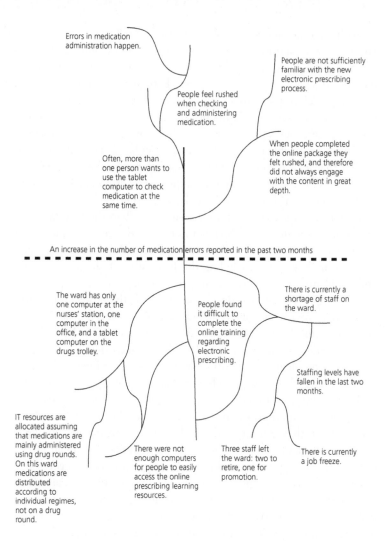

Figure 2.2 Problem Tree analysis: why has there been an increase in the number of medication errors reported in the past two months?

This could, however, be because the computer hardware provided to wards assumes that medication is administered during drug rounds, whereas the ward in question personalizes the timings of drug admin-istration and does not perform a drug round (a 'shared beliefs/values' issue). The Seven S model would therefore need to link the 'structure' problem of inadequate computer hardware with the 'shared beliefs/ values' issue of the importance of individualized care. Otherwise, the real reason why the hardware provided is not adequate would not be clear and might therefore not be addressed in a useful way.

Although the process of problem analysis can be very useful to give an overview of and indications about the causes and effects of a situation, no one approach can, of itself, include or explain all the complexities of every aspect of a problem (European Commission 2004). Each approach to problem analysis has strengths and limitations. The Five Whys analysis and Fishbone Diagram do not easily allow the links between causes to be shown, and rely on the cause, or causes, of a problem being able to be fairly neatly articulated. They also tend to suggest that a clear root cause or causes that can be directly linked to a solution exist, which is not always the case (Latino 2004). Problem Tree analysis can show more links between the potentially complex and interrelated causes of a problem situation than the Five Whys or Fishbone Diagram can, although illustrating the real complexity of any problem will always be difficult to achieve. A limitation of many problem analysis tools, including the Five Whys, Fishbone Diagram, and Problem Tree analysis, is that they do not give prompts about what it might be useful to consider in analysing the problem. For this, a tool that provides specific prompts, such as the Seven S model, can be more useful. However, a downside of the Seven S model is that it may not guide the questioner to look in as much depth at the root causes of a problem as some other approaches do, and may not create such a clear pathway to considering solutions. The problem analysis tools available are intended to guide and enable those confronted with problem situations to unpick and consider the causes and effects involved, but they cannot, of themselves, fully identify the complexities of, or solutions to, any particular problem in practice. Their intention is to encourage individuals and teams to look beyond the superficial, or assumed, problem to ensure that alternative causes are considered. By so doing, they should enable the potentially numerous and interlinked reasons for problems occurring to be identified, which has been highlighted as lacking in many root cause analyses (Keating and Tocco 2013). These processes are, however, most effective when skilled facilitation is available to ensure that alternative explanations for the assumed causes are considered, and that the apparent causes to problems are explored in sufficient depth (Kohfeldt and Langhaut 2012; Keating and Tocco 2013).

2.2.3 The value of using literature review methodology to seek a solution to a problem in practice

Having analysed a problem, and identified its root cause or causes, it is then necessary to seek a solution that addresses these. At this point, literature review methodology can be a useful way to ascertain what is already known about the best way to address the cause or causes of the problem. Using a problem analysis tool might, for instance, have demonstrated that an increase in medication administration errors following the introduction of electronic prescribing was attributable to the required training being insufficient. It might then be useful to carry out a review of the literature to explore the best way to enable healthcare professionals to learn about using electronic prescribing, and the best way of assessing competence in this area. Possible literature review questions might be: 'What is the best way to enable healthcare professionals to learn about electronic prescribing?' or 'What is the most effective way to assess nurses' knowledge about electronic prescribing?'

Identifying and analysing any problem that has presented in practice is, therefore, a necessary precursor to enabling relevant evidence to be sought as a part of addressing it. Nonetheless, whilst literature review methodology may be a useful element of addressing problems in practice, it can also be a valuable part of enabling existing good practice to be maintained and further developed.

2.3 Using a literature review as a part of continuing to develop good practice

Whilst problems are often cited as the reason for developments in practice being needed, it is equally important to recognize, sustain and build on good practice. Unless what works well is cherished and developed, valuable elements of practice are likely to be lost over time. In terms of maintaining and developing people's motivation, it is also vital for the good work and achievements of individuals and teams to be recognized, and valued. Even in situations where the quality of care requires improvement, it has been suggested that this may be best achieved by identifying what individuals and organizations do well, and how this can be used to improve and develop practice, rather than focusing on what is wrong (Moore 2008; Parish 2012). In order to achieve high-quality care it can, therefore, be just as important to identify what currently works well, what people are good at, why this is, and what can be done to sustain and further perfect it, as to identify and solve problems. This can enable individuals and teams to value themselves, their colleagues, their attributes, and to look at how their assets can be used for the purpose of ongoing development rather than blaming one another for any perceived problems (Moore 2008; Parish 2012). One of the ways of beginning the process of identifying and developing ways of building on good practice is to use the principles of appreciative inquiry (Moore 2008; Parish 2012).

2.3.1 Appreciative inquiry

Appreciative inquiry has been used as an approach to both research and organizational development (Kung *et al.* 2013). It is based on the assumption that all individuals and organizations have positive attributes and areas in which they are effective and successful. Appreciative inquiry also acknowledges that there will always be areas of practice in which individuals and organizations could improve what they do. However, it focuses on ensuring that the efforts that have been made, and the skills and strengths of individuals and organizations, are not devalued, missed or lost (Moore 2008; Walsh *et al.* 2009). By recognizing and focusing on these as the basis for enhancing practice, appreciative inquiry uses what is positive within individuals and organizations to counter any negative attributes or problems (Reed 2007; Moore 2008; Koster and Lemelin 2009; Parish 2012). Appreciative inquiry is, therefore, intended to enable individuals and teams to creatively construct a positive future, based on their strengths, and what they value (Moore 2008).

> **Pitfall to avoid**
>
> Do not think that developing practice is always about identifying and resolving problems or areas of deficit: practice can equally be developed by identifying what is currently done well, and should be sustained or further developed.

Using appreciative inquiry to develop practice is, then, a process based on positive recognition of what a team does well, as opposed to a requirement to identify and correct faults. For example, if a team that provides community-based care is considering ways in which to enhance their work using problem-based thinking, they might look at the areas of practice in which they have been found wanting. This could include revisiting any complaints that they have received, or errors that have been made, to identify what problems exist, and how they can seek to remedy these. In contrast, if they seek to identify their strengths, using the principles of appreciative inquiry, they could look at: the compliments they have received; what they feel works well in what they do as individuals and as a team; what they value; and what the people for whom they provide care value. This could enable them to consider ways in which to ensure that these aspects of practice are maintained, and developed even further.

The process of appreciative inquiry is described as having four phases: discovery, dream, design and destiny (often referred to as the 4D Cycle) (Carter *et al.* 2007; Cooperrider *et al.* 2008: 5). It begins with the discovery phase, in which the people concerned describe what they value, find satisfying, or are proud of, in their current work (Cooperrider and Whitney 1999; Cooperrider *et al.* 2008: 5). In the case of the team described above, this phase might lead them to discover that one of the things that they value is knowing the people to whom they provide care as individuals, and thus being able to personalize their care. They might be proud of the fact that, despite the pressures on them, people appreciate their desire to adapt care to each individual's particular needs and preferences. They might also value the loyalty and support that the team give each other, and the respect they have for one another's skills and ideas. This could form a basis from which they develop visions of how things could become even better (Reed 2007; Koster and Lemelin 2009): the second, or 'dream', phase of appreciative inquiry.

In the dream phase of appreciative inquiry, insights into what enables the things that people value, find satisfying, or are proud of in their current work to exist are sought. This step is intended to assist the group to use this information to produce a 'dream' of what they would ideally like to do and be (Cooperrider and Whitney 1999; Cooperrider *et al.* 2008: 5). For the team in question, this could include identifying what it is that enables them to get to know people as individuals and to provide care in a way that matches their particular preferences, despite the pressures of work. Using this process, the team might uncover the importance of them sharing a strongly felt core value concerning the importance of getting to know the people to whom they provide care. They might also realize that because of this they make a deliberate effort to organize their work there so as to achieve as much continuity of care as possible. This positive point might be something that the team could use to ask the dream question: 'Where would we like to take this aspect of our practice, if there were no constraints on us?'

Whilst appreciative inquiry as a whole has to be a grounded in reality, encouraging people to think about what would be their ideal, if there were no restrictions or constraints, can be a useful part of developing the best possible practice. It encourages individuals and teams to see beyond assumed barriers and to think creatively about what could be achieved (Cooperrider and Whitney 1999; Cooperrider *et al.* 2008: 5). For example, the team described here might develop a 'dream' that they would have one member of staff allocated to provide all the care or support that each person needed. This ideal would, of course, not be realistic, because each staff member would have days off and holidays, and thus a person who required daily care for a period of time could not have the same staff member visit to provide that care on every occasion. However, if the team agreed that this was their 'dream' they could explore ways in which they could work to achieve something as close as possible to this, within the realms of possibility.

The third, or 'design', phase of appreciative inquiry focuses on designing how the 'dream' could become a reality. At this point, literature review methodology can be a useful part of the process, as it can enable a team to explore ways in which others have achieved, or tried to achieve, what they aspire to. The existing evidence on the subject can then be used to aid discussions concerning how the 'dream' might be achieved and sustained. If the community care team decided that they wanted to do everything possible to minimize the number of different staff who provided care for each person they might use literature review methodology to ascertain how other teams had tried to achieve this. This might assist them in designing ways to make their 'dream' become a continued reality.

Pitfall to avoid

Do not be afraid to imagine what your ideal would be, if there were no restrictions or constraints. You can use this to develop the best possible option within real world constraints.

The destiny phase of appreciative inquiry focuses on implementing and sustaining the plans and strategies that have been agreed in the design phase (Cooperrider and Whitney 1999; Cooperrider *et al.* 2008: 5; Naude *et al.* 2014). This phase can, and ultimately should, also lead to the development of further discovery, dream and design phases, so that good practice continues to be honed and extended.

2.3.2 Providing evidence to support good practice

As well as being used as a part of an approach such as appreciative inquiry, literature review methodology can also facilitate the provision of evidence to support the need for continued investment in that which facilitates good practice. In a climate in which there are ever-increasing demands on finite resources, it may be very useful to have evidence from the literature to support requests for resources to be retained, or obtained, to enable a team to continue to do what it knows works well. Thus, as well as using literature review methodology to determine how to further develop good practice, it can be a useful tool for demonstrating the worth of what you know from experience works well. For instance, the team providing community-based care might identify that one of the things that enables them to provide good quality care, as perceived by recipients of their service, is continuity of visits, but that this is difficult to achieve without adequate staffing levels. Carrying out a review of the literature might indicate that others have also found this to be the case, providing the team with concrete evidence to support any objection to staffing level cuts.

Summary

Literature review methodology enables the composite evidence on a particular topic to be identified, and, as such, it is particularly useful for answering questions related to what the current best evidence regarding a particular practice issue is. Literature review can be a very useful methodological choice for completing the dissertation requirement for a programme of academic study, as it enables the existing evidence on a subject to be rigorously identified and evaluated. It can also be a valuable part of seeking solutions to problems in practice, provided that these problems are first clearly identified, and their causes determined. In addition, literature review methodology can play a part in exploring ideas about how to sustain and develop what currently works well, and to provide evidence regarding the resources needed to maintain good practice.

Nonetheless, despite being useful in a number of circumstances, a literature review will only make a valuable contribution to knowledge and practice if it is a good quality review.

Appreciative inquiry: an approach to organizational development that is based on the assumption that all individuals and organizations have positive attributes and areas in which they are effective and successful.

Fishbone Diagram: an approach to problem analysis that documents problems and their possible causes by depicting them as a fish skeleton.

Five Whys: an approach to problem analysis that seeks to establish the cause or causes of a problem by asking 'why' questions about it until the root cause or causes of the problem are found.

Problem Tree analysis: an approach to problem analysis that uses the image of a tree to structure and illustrate the exploration of a problem, with the causes of the problem shown as the roots and the effects as the branches.

Seven S model: an approach to problem analysis that maps out the key elements of a team or organization, the roles these may play in a problem situation, and how they interact with each other.

Key points:

- A study that uses literature review methodology should fulfil the requirements of research in terms of being systematic, rigorous and unbiased.
- Steps should be taken to ensure that the review of the literature is conducted without bias.
- To achieve system and rigour, a study that uses literature review methodology must include certain key stages, which should be carried out in a logical order.
- The reasons for the decisions made in a study that uses literature review methodology should be clearly explained.

As Chapter 1 highlighted, there are different types of literature review, each of which have different intentions. Literature review methodology is a form of secondary research, and, as such, a study that uses this approach should fulfil the quality standards required of research in terms of being rigorous, systematic and free from bias (Cronin *et al.* 2008; Roberts and Bailey 2010; Aveyard 2014: 2–3). Subsequent chapters will discuss how each particular element of a study that uses literature review methodology should be conducted. However, for the review to be deemed to be of good quality, it needs to have a logical, systematic and rigorous thread running throughout it. This will enable the reader to follow the decisions made, the reasons for these being made, and see consistency between the stages of the review. As a result, the review as a whole should be one that they are confident accurately represents reality.

A good literature review enables the reader to easily see how everything in it fits together. In contrast, in a poor quality review, the reader wonders how and why decisions were made, and is distracted by apparent gaps or inconsistencies between the different elements of the review. Therefore, before considering the discrete elements of a study that uses literature review methodology, this chapter outlines the key features of a good review, including: the study being rigorous, systematic, unbiased and explaining the rationale for the decisions taken within it. These principles apply to any study that uses literature review methodology, regardless of the size and scope of the review.

> **Pitfall to avoid**
>
> Make sure that there is a logical progression of ideas between the sections of your literature review, and that the study forms a coherent whole, with no unexplained gaps or inconsistencies.

3.1 What makes a literature review rigorous?

One of the qualities of good research is that it is rigorous (Pereira 2012; Claydon 2015). Thus, in order to be judged to be a sound piece of research, a study that uses literature review methodology must be conducted rigorously.

Being rigorous can be defined as being 'severely accurate' or 'strict' (Collins Dictionaries 2014). To achieve rigour, each aspect of a study that uses literature review methodology therefore needs to be conducted thoroughly, and carefully, so that the findings are an accurate representation of the existing evidence. To be rigorous, a study that uses literature review methodology must also adhere accurately and strictly to the accepted methodological standards for this type of research. As subsequent chapters discuss, the way in which these standards are met varies slightly, depending on the type of literature being reviewed, and the extent of the review. However, there needs to be evidence of the relevant standards being achieved in order for a review to attain the criteria of rigour. For example, as Chapter 6 discusses, there will always need to be evidence that accepted processes for searching diligently for the existing literature on the subject in question were used (Kamienski et al. 2013; Aveyard 2014: 74; Waltho et al. 2015). In addition, as Chapter 7 outlines, it should always be clear that the literature gathered was evaluated without bias, using criteria or tools that were fit for this purpose (Cronin et al. 2008; Murphy et al. 2009; Aveyard 2014: 110).

Being rigorous does not, however, mean that a review has to cover every aspect of any subject area. As Chapter 5 discusses, it is much better to conduct a review that comprehensively addresses a very specific and clearly focused aspect of a subject than to try to cover a broad topic area, and consequently struggle to achieve the requisite quality standards (Holland 2007; Lipowski 2008; Offredy and Vickers 2010). Rigour is not achieved by a study trying to be all-encompassing, but by it being very explicit about what it does and does not cover, and then fulfilling this remit. You might, for example, be interested in exploring the evidence about the support provided to young people who are at risk of suicide, and their families. However, conducting a rigorous review of the evidence on this entire subject area would be difficult to achieve, especially if the study was being undertaken for your dissertation. As Chapter 5 discusses, the more focused the review question, and by implication the less breadth it seeks to cover, the more rigorous the review tends to be. In this instance, you might decide to focus your review on the evidence concerning the best way to support parents whose children are at risk of suicide. This would, of course, mean that some aspects of your broad area of interest were not included. However, the quality of the study you undertook would be likely to benefit from this decision in terms of it being rigorous, systematic and focused.

Pitfall to avoid

Do not try to cover every aspect of a subject area in your review. The more focused your review, the more likely it is to be rigorous.

Rigour is an important quality standard for a study that uses literature review methodology to achieve. However, in order to be a good quality review, the study must also be systematic.

3.2 What makes a study that uses literature review methodology systematic?

Being systematic means being 'characterized by the use of order and planning' or 'methodical' (Collins Dictionaries 2014). A literature review being systematic is intrinsically linked with it achieving rigour, because if everything is planned and carried out in an orderly and methodical fashion, the study is more likely to be rigorous. A study being systematic requires everything in it to be planned and undertaken in a manner that means that nothing is missed out, and that each stage in the review process proceeds logically to the next. For example, in order to be systematic, a literature review needs to arrive at a clearly formulated question before planning the methodological steps that need to be taken in order to address this question. If the review's methodological steps are planned or commenced before the question is clear, there is a risk that the literature that is collected will not all be relevant to the focus of the review, and that important evidence will be omitted. This will detract from the system of the study, and in turn affect its rigor.

Being systematic also means that the way in which the review is conducted is logical and that there is consistency between its stages. There should, for instance, as Chapters 4 and 5 discuss, be a clear indication of why the review was undertaken that logically leads to the question or questions that are addressed in the review. The aims and objectives of the review should, as Chapter 5 outlines, then follow on from the study question. The methods used to locate relevant literature should be commensurate with addressing these aims and answering the review question. These methods should be clearly explained, and accompanied by the reasons for the decisions that were made concerning them. After explaining how the literature to be reviewed was gathered, the results from the search should be stated, including the final number of papers included in the review, and how these were selected. This degree of clarity enables the reader to feel confident that relevant literature was searched for diligently, and thoroughly, in accordance with clearly defined decisions. It also provides assurances that no relevant evidence was inadvertently omitted, or any irrelevant material erroneously included, because of chance, errors or bias (Cronin *et al.* 2008; Aveyard 2014: 3–4).

The way in which the literature was evaluated should then be explained, with a rationale given for the selection of any tools that were used to perform this appraisal. This stage should convince the reader that all the evidence was appraised methodically, carefully and without bias. The appraisal of each individual paper should, as Chapter 8 describes, be followed by an explanation of how the information gathered from this stage of the review was synthesized to determine the composite evidence from across sources.

The findings from this synthesis of the evidence should be linked back to the study question, providing answers to this, and to the aims, showing how they were addressed. If the findings do not enable the study question to be answered, then there is a fault in review process. The answer to the review question may be one that enables very specific conclusions for best practice to be made. Equally, though, the answer may be that there is currently insufficient or inconsistent evidence regarding, for example, the best way to support the parents of young people who are at risk of suicide. However, it should be clear to the reader that the review question was addressed, using a systematic and rigorous process, even if this process showed that the current evidence on the subject is inconclusive.

> **Pitfall to avoid**
>
> Do not view your review as a series of unconnected stages. The stages of the review should be logically linked, and have a consistent thread of decision-making running through them.

To be systematic, a literature review must therefore have no unexplained gaps in its process, and the process used should follow a logical and efficient order. This enables the reader to feel convinced that the findings could not have been subject to bias by any information being omitted or misinterpreted.

3.3 Bias

A hallmark of good quality research is that it is unbiased. However, how the issue of bias is addressed in a study is in part dependent on the nature of the research in question. In a study that uses literature review methodology, it means that the opinions, views or preconceptions of the reviewer do not influence how the study is conducted or their interpretation of the existing literature on the subject being investigated. The person conducting the review needs to be open to the question that they pose receiving any answer, and to avoid trying to make the evidence fit a particular point that they wish to make. For example, if you work in child and adolescent mental health services, and are interested in conducting a literature review on the best way to support families whose children display suicidal tendencies, the likelihood is that you will have experience, views and opinions regarding this. These may be gained from practice and from what you have read. However, if your review is intended to answer the question: 'What is the best way to support parents whose children are at risk of suicide?' the answer has to be able to be whatever a rigorous and systematic review of the existing literature suggests, even if it is at odds with what you expected, hoped it would be, or thought it should be.

> **Pitfall to avoid**
>
> Avoid suggesting you knew the answer to the review question before carrying out your study.

In addition be being unbiased in your thinking, the way you present your review needs to convince your reader of your neutrality. One way of achieving this is to explicitly state the rationale for the decisions that you make. This enables the reader to understand why you made the decisions that you did, and to see that these were based on sound principles, not personal preferences that could bias or skew the study's findings.

3.4 Providing a rationale for decisions

Conducting a study that uses literature review methodology involves making a number of decisions, and the reasoning behind these decisions should be clear in your study report. If you decided to focus your review on the best way to support parents whose children are at risk of suicide, you would need to explain why you chose this focus, so as to convince your reader that there was a good reason for your decision. The reader does not necessarily need to agree with your choices, because in many cases there is no one right decision. In the case of deciding which aspect of the evidence concerning the support provided to young people who are at risk of suicide, and their families, should be explored, there would be many perfectly good choices that could be made. Your task is not to demonstrate that yours was the only right choice, but to convince your reader that you made a perfectly reasonable, and reasoned, decision.

In terms of methodological choices, the same principle applies: these should be shown to be well thought out and justifiable. For instance, as Chapter 6 discusses, a variety of tools exist that can be used to evaluate different types of evidence, and there is not complete agreement as to which tool is the best to use in any particular circumstance. Your task, as the person conducting and presenting the review, is to explain why you chose the tool or tools that you did, including what you understand the strengths and limitations of your decision to be. Providing your reader with this level of information helps to guard against concerns about bias by making the process of your decision-making transparent.

Your decisions being clear will also help to convince your reader that you have been rigorous. It demonstrates that you have not simply done things for convenience, by chance, or without thinking of the consequences that your actions will have on the quality of your review. Instead, it demonstrates that there was a sound and well-thought-out reason for everything that you did, which contributes to achieving the criteria of being systematic in terms of the study being orderly, well planned and methodical. This clarity over decision-making processes should be evident in each element of the review, but there should also be consistency of decision-making between each of the key aspects of the study.

Pitfall to avoid

Do not assume that the reasons for your decisions will be obvious to your reader. In most circumstances, providing a clear explanation for your decisions will enhance your review.

3.5 The key elements of literature review methodology

For a review of the literature to be rigorous and systematic, certain processes must be included in it, and these should be performed in a logical order. The elements that must be included in any study that uses literature review methodology form the content of the individual chapters in the next section of this book. However, an overview of what these should be, and their sequence, is as follows:

A study that uses literature review methodology should usually begin by presenting a background to the review, and a rationale for it being performed. These sections should provide the reader with a focused discussion of what led you to carry out the review, and why you have focused on the area that you have (Levy and Ellis 2006; Denscombe 2012). This should take the reader to a point from which the study question, aims and objectives naturally follow.

There needs to be a clear link between the background to the study, the reasons you have given for undertaking the study, and the study question and aims. For example, if the background and rationale sections of your study focus on the causes of suicide amongst young people, and ways of preventing this, the review question being: 'What is the best way to support the parents of young people who are considered to be at risk of suicide?' is not a logical next step. There is, of course, a link between suicide prevention in young people and providing support for their parents, and your reader could probably work out what this is, but they would have to do this: you have not led them to it. Your job as the writer of the review is to lead the reader directly to your question, not to provide detailed hints and then expect them to find their own way to it. Thus, if your review question is about the support provided for parents, your background information needs to lead your reader directly to why this is important, relevant, and the reason that you selected it as the focus of your review. Chapter 5 discusses the development of the study question, aims and objectives, but these should be clearly stated and a reasoned culmination of the background and rationale provided for your review. They should also proceed logically from one another, so that, for instance, meeting the aims of the review would allow the review question to be answered.

> **Pitfall to avoid**
>
> Avoid having unexplained gaps in the flow of ideas or inconsistencies in the decisions made between the sections of your study report.

Having set the scene for the study, and clarified through the review question, aims and objectives exactly what the study explores, the next stage of the review is the methodology: the way in which literature was sought, evaluated and synthesized. These elements of a literature review are discussed in Chapters 6, 7 and 8, and are the logical next steps because they provide your reader with the details of how literature was gathered, evaluated and synthesized in order to address the review aims and answer the study question. These stages should appear after the study background, rationale, question, aims and objectives because your reader needs to know what you intended to study before they know how you studied it. In addition, some of the decisions concerning the methodology of the review are dependent on what was decided in the preceding sections. For example, if one of the study aims was to review the evidence regarding parents' perceptions of the support they need, you might have decided that it was appropriate to use evidence from both qualitative and quantitative research. Your rationale for this decision might have been: quantitative research would allow numerical evidence about how parents rate the quality of particular services to be determined, but qualitative research would also be important to gain an in-depth understanding of parents' views and experiences. For a review to be considered systematic, the decisions made in the methodology need to be consistent with the study's question, aims and objectives, and the logic behind these decisions must be clear.

The methodology outlines how the review of the literature was conducted, and should therefore be followed by the findings from that review. As Chapters 7 and 8 discuss, the findings should include how much relevant literature was found, where it was found, and the nature and strength of that evidence. Exactly how the findings section is arranged will, as Chapters 7 and 8 discuss, depend on a number of factors, but the findings must meet the study aims and answer the review question. For example, if the review question was: 'What is the best way to provide support for the parents of young people who are at risk of suicide?' the findings should all relate to this issue. They should, as with any research, also be a logical culmination of the methodological decisions that have been stated. If the methodology stated that only evidence from quantitative research was sought, the findings should only present a review of the quantitative evidence. If both qualitative and quantitative research were included, both types of evidence should feature in the findings.

The findings from the review should be followed by a discussion of these findings. Chapter 8 explores approaches to structuring the discussion of the findings, and highlights that, whilst there must be a logical flow between the findings from the review and the discussion of these, the discussion should not simply restate the findings (Lunenburg and Irby 2008; White 2011). It should, rather, enter into a critical analysis of the findings, including an evaluation of ways in which these corroborate, build on or differ from other evidence on the subject (Lunenburg and Irby 2008; White 2011). Whilst the discussion section should explore the findings in some depth, it must only include issues that have been highlighted in the findings (White 2011). It should also be clearly focused on the review's question and aims, so that the study remains systematically focused on these key issues (Lunenburg and Irby 2008; White 2011). The findings from a literature review might, for instance, indicate that all the papers reviewed show good evidence that supporting the parents of young people who are at risk of suicide is an important part of preventing teenage suicide. In this case, the discussion of this finding might include whether this belief is apparent in existing recommendations or guidelines, and why this might be so. However the discussion, whilst encompassing wider evidence and commentary, would still be focused around something that was found in the review, and that addressed the study question.

Pitfall to avoid

Do not include issues in the discussion of the findings from your review that did not feature in the findings themselves.

The discussion section of the review should be followed by the conclusions and recommendations that can be drawn from the study.

These must be based on the findings, answer the study question, and show that the aims have been addressed (Lunenburg and Irby 2008; White 2011). A finding from a review might be that there is good evidence that supporting the parents of young people who are thought to be at risk of suicide is an important part of reducing the incidence of teenage suicide. In this case, the conclusions could reasonably include that the parents of young people who are at risk of suicide should be provided with support. The recommendations might then include that healthcare providers explore how funding can be made available for parents to be supported. These would be a logical conclusion and recommendation arising from the study. However, to deviate into what might be the barriers to funding being made available, and how these could be overcome, would be inappropriate at this stage of the study. Unless it was a part of the remit of the review, and had featured in the findings, it would not be a recommendation that could be made because of the review of the literature. For a study that uses literature review methodology to be rigorous, systematic and unbiased the conclusions and recommendations made must arise from the findings (White 2011).

A study that uses literature review methodology should, like any research, include a discussion of the strengths and limitations of the study, and their effect on the findings, conclusions and recommendations (Murray 2011; White 2011). These issues may, as Chapters 8 and 9 highlight, be presented as a part of the discussion, or as a separate section, but their effect on the study should be clear. The strength or confidence with which the conclusions and recommendations are stated should, as Chapter 10 outlines, be consistent with the strengths and limitations of the review. As a result, the claims made should be identifiably commensurate with the strength of the evidence derived from the review.

Pitfall to avoid

Avoid making conclusions or recommendations that are either over- or understated in relation to the strength of the evidence from the review.

Summary

Being rigorous, systematic and unbiased are important quality indicators in any research, including studies that use literature review methodology. Achieving these standards means that what the review presents can be trusted to be an accurate representation of the existing evidence on a subject. It means that nothing that the review claimed to cover was missed out, that the judgements made were based on an unbiased examination of the available evidence, and that there were no process errors that might have led to the findings, conclusions or recommendations being inaccurate. These qualities mean that the reader can confidently act on the findings from the review.

Part II of this book will now discuss each of the key stages of a study that uses literature review methodology, and how they should be conducted and presented.

> ## Terminology
>
> **Bias:** 'a mental tendency or inclination, especially an irrational preference or prejudice' (Collins Dictionaries 2014). A literature review being biased would mean that the review was influenced by the reviewer's inclinations, preferences or prejudices, rather than being based around sound methodological decisions and judgements.
>
> **Rigorous:** 'severely accurate' or 'strict' (Collins Dictionaries 2014). A rigorous literature review should be conducted thoroughly, carefully, and strictly adhere to the accepted methodological standards for this type of research.
>
> **Systematic:** 'characterized by the use of order and planning' or 'methodical' (Collins Dictionaries 2014). For a literature review to be systematic, everything in it should be planned and carried out in an orderly manner so that nothing is omitted, and each stage in the review process proceeds logically to the next.

Key points:

- A study that uses literature review methodology should begin by presenting a background and rationale that identify why the review was undertaken.
- The background should critically and analytically present contextual literature that sets the scene for the review and identifies why it is needed.
- The rationale should explore reasons other than those presented in the background section that have led to the study being undertaken.
- The background and rationale should lead the reader logically to the study question and aims.

The background and rationale that you provide for your literature review should enable the reader to understand what the review will be about, and why you decided to undertake it (Denscombe 2012). The person reading your study may be very familiar with your subject area, or they may know very little about it. The background and rationale should therefore be written in a way that enables anyone, regardless of their expertise in the field, to follow your line of argument, understand your explanations, and be clear about what has led you to your study question and aims. For example, you may have decided to carry out a literature review on the best way to manage women's pain immediately post hysterectomy. In this case, after reading the background and rationale for the review the reader should, regardless of their professional background, understand why this subject matters, what your exact focus will be, and why literature review methodology is an appropriate approach to take. A good quality background and rationale therefore allow a non-expert to understand what a review will be about, and why it is needed, even if they do not understand the medical or technical details of what is discussed.

Pitfall to avoid

Do not assume that your reader will be familiar with your subject.

4.1 Writing the background for a study that uses literature review methodology

Quick and Hall (2015) suggest that carrying out a critical appraisal of the current evidence on your chosen topic is one of the most important stages of any study. It enables you to demonstrate that you understand not only your particular subject area, but also the wider context into which your study fits, and therefore why you have selected to focus on the specific area that you have (Boote and Beile 2005; Levy and Ellis 2006). This begins the task of convincing your reader that you have been systematic and rigorous in your enquiry, have not made any assumptions about what is and is not already known, and can justify your decisions (Boote and Beile 2005; Levy and Ellis 2006). First impressions count in every walk of life, and the background and rationale that you present for your study will be an important first impression for your reader.

If you carry out a literature review without first exploring the current evidence on the subject in question, there is a risk that you will duplicate existing knowledge, miss the opportunity to fill a significant gap in what is known, or embark on a piece of work that will be unachievable (Tungpunkom and Turale 2014). By analysing the existing information about a subject, and the ways in which it has already been investigated, you should be able to ensure that your study is necessary, and that you are using the best approach to developing knowledge in your chosen field. For example, if you were interested in investigating the best way to manage pain immediately post hysterectomy, you might find that a lot of research had already been conducted in this area, but that the studies seemed to have slightly different findings or recommendations. This would suggest a possible gap in knowledge about what the composite evidence regarding the best way to manage pain immediately post hysterectomy was. A study that used literature review methodology would, in this case, seem to be an appropriate way to fill this gap. In contrast, if you identified that there was no existing research on this particular subject, it would clarify that a study using literature review methodology would be impossible to conduct. In this instance, primary research would be a better way to approach knowledge generation.

If you are carrying out a review of the literature because a number of studies on the subject that you are interested in exist, but there are no recent reviews that clarify the composite best evidence, you should explain this in your study background. Noting this demonstrates that you have checked the existing evidence, confirmed that your review is needed, and why this is. The age of the existing evidence is also worth commenting on in the background to your review. If, for instance, a review of the evidence on your subject has been conducted, but is now ten years old, an updated review would usually be justifiable. This would be especially so if several relevant studies had been published since the previous review. If, on the other hand, a review on exactly the same subject has been conducted within the past year, the need for another one might be less obvious. This does not preclude you from performing such a review, but the rationale for doing so would require clarification: some additional studies might have been published since the initial review, and explaining this would be a task for you to accomplish in the study background. Similarly, a review might exist that includes evidence from North America, Australasia and Europe. If you work in England, you might feel that there are enough specific issues in the United Kingdom (UK) to merit carrying out a review that focuses only on UK-based literature. These decisions, and the reasons behind them, should be clearly articulated, so that your reader can understand what you are planning to do, why there is value in doing it, and can see that the task will be achievable.

> **Pitfall to avoid**
>
> Do not design a study without first diligently checking the existing evidence in your chosen subject area.

4.1.1 Being analytical

Reviewing the background literature on the subject that you want to study is an essential precursor to developing the review question, aims and methodology. However, to be a good quality argument for undertaking the review, the background needs to go beyond presenting the literature on your chosen subject. In most walks of life, very little credibility is attached to those who claim to know about something, but are subsequently found to have very limited insight into the subject. Much more credibility is attached to those who demonstrate that they have sought out a range of information, opinions and experiences, and can show considered and thoughtful analysis of these. Similarly, deciding to carry out a literature review without first ensuring, and convincing others, that you have sought out and critically considered the existing evidence will not make your study credible. In contrast, showing that you have diligently considered all the viewpoints and evidence on a subject will begin the process of convincing your reader that you have a sound knowledge of the topic under investigation, and can be trusted to investigate it rigorously, systematically and without bias. Therefore, as well as developing a clear argument in your background, you need to show a degree of critical analysis of what has (and has not) already been written on the subject in question (Boote and Beile 2005).

Your task in the study background is, then, to faithfully, but critically, represent the existing evidence. To achieve this, you should analytically identify not only what is written on the subject, but also the differences in findings between studies, variations of opinions between authors, and the gaps in what is known. Being critical in this context does not mean being negative: it means showing the ability to appreciate the existing work in the field, its strengths, limitations, focus and intended application. This enables you to explain not only the quality and purpose of individual pieces of evidence, but to demonstrate the extent of the existing evidence base as a whole, the significance of this, and its importance for your study (Davey 2007; Denscombe 2012; Quick and Hall 2015). Box 4.1 shows an example of how critical consideration of the background literature could be used to inform the development of a study that uses literature review methodology.

Pitfall to avoid

Avoid presenting a description of the existing evidence without critically evaluating its quality, application and how this has led you to undertake your chosen study.

Demonstrating that you have engaged in a critical evaluation of the existing evidence enables you to reduce the chance of your work being, or seeming, biased. As you explore the background literature that informs your review, ensuring that you include evidence or opinions that are at odds with either your own ideas or the dominant views enables you to think more widely, and question assumptions. It also allows you to demonstrate to your reader that you did this, were open to a range of views, and that your review is based on a balanced

Box 4.1

Deciding to carry out a literature review

Lara is interested in exploring the best way to support the families of people who are discharged from hospital following stroke. She has gathered a lot of evidence on this subject, including research, opinion papers, case reports and policies, and has found that whilst there is common ground between these, different documents have slightly different findings, conclusions and recommendations. Her initial thoughts from perusing the existing evidence are that there are a number of research papers on this subject, but that the focus of these varies. Some concern the support that families receive prior to discharge, whilst others focus on the support provided once the person is at home. In addition, some of the research has been conducted with any family members who are caregivers for the person, others are concerned with spouses or partners, whilst one or two include any family members. The age groups studied and degree of residual disability that the person has following stroke also varies between papers. Thus, the intended application of the papers she has differs. The methodology used and the quality of the papers also varies. Identifying and exploring these differences has led Lara to believe that a more in-depth review of the existing evidence will be beneficial, as it appears that there is not complete clarity over what is and is not known on this subject, and what advice applies to which particular group of people. Lara works with older people, and has found that there is a body of research in this area, but no existing review of the overall evidence. She has therefore decided to carry out a study using literature review methodology, to explore the support required by family members of older people who have suffered a stroke, focusing on those who will be involved in the person's ongoing day-to-day care.

argument (Boote and Beile 2005; Denscombe 2012). In contrast, if your background suggests that you have accepted existing ideas, opinions and findings uncritically, or have only considered one side of the argument, your reader may begin to wonder whether your study as a whole will be lacking in rigour, or biased. It may sometimes be the case that there are no dissenting voices to highlight in your discussion. In such instances it is worth explaining this, so that your reader knows that the argument you have presented represents the complete current published perspectives, rather than wondering if you have been selective in your searching or reporting of the literature.

4.1.2 What to include in the review background

The things that may be relevant to include in the background to your review include: the historical context of the subject; policies; theories; perspectives; ideas; issues or problems that make the review necessary; and any definitions that will be used in the review (Denscombe 2012). As well as including these in the background to your study, you need to be able to show the links between them. Sometimes the links will be easy to make, for example, the history of a subject and the development of particular policies related to it may be intertwined. In other cases, you may have to explain these links, and lead your reader through the process of understanding how things fit together, and ultimately lead to your study question and aims. As you develop the links between sections in your background, remember that your reader may have limited knowledge of your particular subject area, so avoid making assumptions or expecting them to make the links between ideas. That is your responsibility as the writer. For example, if you decided to use literature review methodology to explore the evidence concerning the management of pain immediately post hysterectomy, you might begin by presenting a short historical context of how pain has been perceived and managed, culminating in current perceptions, how this has led to the development of ways of measuring or assessing pain, and to policies, guidance and protocols on the management of pain. Whilst many people will be able to make a link between these elements of your discussion, for example between how pain is now perceived and how it is assessed, making these links explicit is your task as the writer.

Pitfall to avoid

Do not expect your reader to make the links between the ideas that you present.

In addition to deciding what to include in your background, and developing the links and logic between elements of your discussion, you will need to make a decision as to how much of your word allowance to devote to each element. As you consider this, remember that you also need to be critically analytical of the existing evidence. Whilst the historical context of any subject can be very important, it is often expedient to avoid a lengthy description of the history of a particular issue that does not provide any analysis or direct links to your review. For example, if you are exploring post hysterectomy pain management, the history of how pain perception has changed over time may be very important to include in the background, so that the reader understands that our current perspectives have not always been the dominant view. However, a lengthy description of historic views on pain and its management will often be more than you have the space to include. You might, perhaps, include a paragraph on how pain and its management have been perceived over time, highlighting key points at which views on managing pain altered. This enables you to continue your discussion by introducing and analysing current perspectives, and to begin the process of funnelling the discussion to your very specific topic area. As you make these decisions, keep in mind where you need to get to, the amount of material you need to cover to get there, what your most important points in a background discussion will be, and what the word limit for your report is.

Pitfall to avoid

Avoid spending a significant part of your word allowance on a purely descriptive account of the historical background to your study.

Whilst the background to your review should focus from a broad area down to a much narrower element of the subject that you plan to study, the overall breadth that you cover will vary, depending on the topic that you are exploring. If you are reviewing the literature on a topic about which very little has been written your background may need to include information from a broad field of enquiry (Boote and Beile 2005). In contrast, if you are reviewing the literature on a topic about which a great deal has been written you may instead need to focus from the start on a fairly narrow field (Boote and Beile 2005). If you were carrying out a literature review regarding post hysterectomy pain management, you might find that relatively little had been written about this subject. In this situation, you might well begin the study background by exploring definitions of pain, the history of pain management, theories of pain management, why pain management is important generally, why it is important post operatively, different approaches to managing post operative pain, their strengths, limitations and the evidence for this. You might then outline the statistics of how many women undergo hysterectomy annually (so as to indicate the importance of this issue), provide a critical overview of the literature on post hysterectomy pain management, and why a review of this literature is needed. On the other hand, you might find that there was a great deal of information, guidance and opinion on post hysterectomy pain management. Your discussion of: the definitions of pain; history of pain management; theories of pain management; why pain management is important generally; why it is important post operatively; different approaches to managing post operative pain; and their strengths, limitations and the evidence for this would, in this situation, need to be more succinct. This would allow you to quickly hone in on post hysterectomy pain management, perhaps dividing this into sections concerning immediate post operative management, management in the first twenty-four hours post surgery, management for different types of hysterectomy, etc., in a manner which took the reader to your focus.

Given the range of decisions that can be made about the background section of your report, it is useful to explain early on in this section what your discussion will include. This allows the reader to understand the key areas that you aim to cover and why you have decided on this, and to see that you were systematic and rigorous in your decision-making. You should try to avoid giving the reader the opportunity to think: 'But you haven't considered…'. Although your background can never include everything ever written that might be relevant to your subject, what the limits of the background discussion will be should be clear, and you should demonstrate that you are aware of any areas that have been intentionally omitted, and have a good reason for excluding them from your discussion.

The background and rationale sections of your literature review are intended to take your reader on a logical journey to the review's question and aims. As Chapter 5 will discuss, the study question and the aims that you develop will be based around certain key terms and concepts. In order to ensure that your reader knows exactly what you plan to explore, you should therefore usually include a definition of the key terms that will be used in the background section of your study. These terms may be open to different interpretations, and providing these definitions enables you to clarify exactly what these will be taken to mean in the context of your study, and how you will be using them. As well as stating your definitions, you should show how these were developed: for example, whether they were drawn from the work of established authorities in the field, and, where there are variations in how the terms are defined, why you have chosen the definition that you have.

There may be instances where you choose, or need, to develop your own definition or definitions. In such situations, you should explain why this was the case and, in order to justify your decision, discuss the alternative choices that you could have made, and the reasons why you do not make these (Denscombe 2012). The definitions used in your review should, therefore, be presented clearly, with a sound rationale for the choices you made, and thereafter be rigorously and systematically applied throughout your work.

As a whole, the study background should present a logical, analytical evaluation of the background to your review, and, by so doing, justify why the study was undertaken.

4.2 The distinction between the discussion of the background literature and the detailed review and synthesis of individual papers

The question often arises in studies that use literature review methodology as to the difference between the background literature that informs the review, and the selection and analysis of the studies that are included in the review itself (as outlined in Chapters 6, 7 and 8). The distinction is that in the background section the literature is much broader: it sets the scene for the study and shows why the review is needed. To this end, it includes a wider range of information than the papers that are used for the purpose of data collection and analysis as described in Chapters 7 and 8. Although it provides a background discussion and analysis of why a review of the current evidence on a subject is important, the background section does not present an in-depth, study-by-study review of that evidence.

Whilst the background section of a literature review does not include the step-by-step, rigorous appraisal of individual papers that is undertaken for the main part of the review, at least some of those papers are likely to feature in it. For example, if you intend to use literature review methodology to conduct a study on the best way to manage women's pain in the first twenty-four hours post hysterectomy, your review papers will all be focused on this exact subject. However, the study background, as the previous sections of this chapter have discussed, will use information drawn from a much broader topic area than this, and will end more or less at the beginning point of the review itself. Some of the literature that you use in the latter part of the background to the review will, however, usually also be included in the review itself. The distinction between how these papers are situated in these sections is that in the background they are highlighted, and what seem to be their key strengths, limitations, differences and similarities are discussed. This is accompanied by an explanation of why these initial impressions make it seem useful to review the literature in greater depth in order to identify the current best evidence.

The background to the study therefore includes both the broad literature around your subject area and some very specific literature related to the exact focus of your review. As a result, it should take your reader on a clear journey to why you are undertaking the review in question.

> **Pitfall to avoid**
>
> Do not use the study background to rehearse your main review.

The background to a study that uses literature review methodology provides a literature-based justification for conducting the review. In addition, a rationale for the study that covers reasons other than the existing literature-based evidence for conducting the review is generally useful to include.

4.3 The rationale for the study

The rationale for your review should form a logical continuation from the background literature, but is about why, apart from the literature that you have already outlined, you decided to conduct the review, in terms of both subject area and methodology. The content of this section will therefore depend on why you have become interested in undertaking the review. It may have some overlaps with the background and, in this case, you should be careful not to repeat yourself, and may need to make a decision as to which section some aspects of your discussion will best fit.

There is a strong likelihood that a part of your rationale for undertaking the review will be what you have seen and experienced in practice, and what your role in practice is (even if you are undertaking your literature review as part of a programme of study). As Chapter 2 identifies, a literature review may sometimes be designed to address a problem in practice, or to develop and further hone an area of good practice. If this is the case, such issues should be highlighted in the rationale, and how the focus of the review was decided upon outlined, so that the reader can see the steps that were taken to ensure that you were addressing the right area for development or problem resolution (Denscombe 2012). This discussion of how you determined what your focus would be is a part of demonstrating that your study is based on a systematic and rigorous process. Presenting any practice-based need for your review in a rigorous and systematic manner adds to the impression of diligence, system and rigour in the study as a whole.

As you discuss how you reached any practice-based rationale for your study, you should not, as with the background literature, expect your reader to make the necessary links between ideas. For instance, a process of appreciative inquiry (as described in Chapter 2) may have led you to decide to use literature review methodology to explore the best way to manage women's pain in the first twenty-four hours post hysterectomy. In this case, you should outline in the rationale for your study what led you to this decision. This might include a discussion of what you and your colleagues feel you do well and value in your current practice, including the value you attach to ensuring that women are pain free post surgery. This, alongside the fact that your discussions were conducted on a gynaecology ward, might seem to provide a perfect rationale for your review. However, it would be useful to state the links between ideas more clearly to your reader. You could explain that whilst good pain control is something that is valued, and generally appears to be achieved in your workplace, the ward team identified that they wanted to be more certain that they were using the best possible methods of pain control, particularly in the immediate post operative period. For this reason, a review of the literature was seen as potentially useful in taking practice to an even higher level, in terms of the evidence on which it was based. This type of small linking explanation can enable your reader to follow your logic, to understand exactly what you aimed to explore, and why you made the decisions that you did.

Your rationale might also be concerned with the policy that informs practice and thus have some overlap with the background. For example, if there is local, national or international guidance on a particular practice issue that is being implemented in your workplace, you may be seeking to evaluate the evidence behind this policy, or the best way to implement it. Equally you might be in a position where you need to develop guidance for use in practice and want to carry out a review of the literature to ensure that what you produce is based on the current best evidence. These reasons for undertaking the review of the literature would not only have subject-based rationales, but also methodological rationales, as they would provide a clear reason for using literature review methodology.

Pitfall to avoid

Remember to include both methodological and subject-based reasons for conducting your review throughout the background and rationale to the study.

Another practice-based rationale for your review might be that the people whom you work with have different perspectives on the best way to manage a clinical issue, such as post hysterectomy pain. If the background literature also indicates that there are several different perspectives on this, your reason for conducting a literature review might be the need for clarity over what the composite best evidence actually is, so as to be able to reduce confusion and inconsistencies in practice. Again, this provides a practice-based subject and methodological reason for the review being necessary.

Closely linked to the practice-based rationale for your study, it is likely that you will have a professional interest in the subject that you have selected for your literature review. A part of your rationale may therefore be to discuss your own professional interest in the area. For example, if you are the link nurse for pain management on a gynaecology ward, then your interest in reviewing the literature on pain management immediately post hysterectomy would probably be associated with that role. Alternatively, the subject that you have chosen to review may not be linked with an official role, but be something you are interested in and want to learn more about. For instance, if you have recently begun working on a gynaecology ward you may be interested in understanding more about the optimum way to manage post operative pain in women who have undergone hysterectomy, and your dissertation may be a good opportunity to explore this. Equally, you may be studying a subject that is not linked to your current practice. It may be that you hope to work in a particular area in the future, and want to take the opportunity to learn more about this.

The rationale section of your literature review can, therefore, include a number of issues, depending on what has led you to undertake your study. Box 4.2 shows an example of things that might be included in a study rationale. However, like the background section, these should be presented logically and analytically, and demonstrate a lack of bias. If, for instance, your rationale indicates that you have identified different approaches to managing pain post hysterectomy, and want to explore the best way forward, it should also demonstrate that you are open-minded about what the review will find this to be.

Box 4.2

The rationale for the review

A study rationale may include:

- practice-based reasons:

  - seeking a solution to a problem in practice;
  - development of best practice;
  - identification of the ideal for best practice;
  - clarification over differences in opinion over the best approach to practice;
  - a need to implement guidance for practice;
  - a need to develop guidelines for practice.

- methodological reasons:

  - there is a range of evidence on the subject in question but no existing review that draws all this together;
  - people cite different evidence to justify different approaches to practice: there is therefore a need to clarify what the existing evidence really says.

- professional interest
- personal interest

Pitfall to avoid

Avoid suggesting that the rationale for undertaking your review is to prove a particular point.

Summary

As Chapter 3 highlighted, one of the characteristics of any high-quality study is there being a logical and consistent link between its sections, and evidence of rigour and system throughout the process of enquiry. The background and rationale sections of a study that uses literature review methodology begin this process. After reading the background and rationale to the review your reader should have an understanding of the breadth of the subject area that your study is located within, why you have chosen the focus you have, and how your study fits within the existing evidence base. These sections should also demonstrate that, whilst you have an interest in the subject, your study will be conducted impartially. The background and rationale for your study should lead logically to your study question and aims.

Key points:

- The review question should be clear, focused and achievable.
- The aims of the review should set out what the study intends to accomplish, and their achievement should mean that the study question is answered.
- The objectives of the review should detail how the aims will be achieved. As such they should be actions that directly link to the aims.
- The review question, aims and objectives should all clearly relate to one another.

Having a clear and focused question, aims and objectives for your literature review are important steps towards your study as a whole being rigorous and systematic (Cronin *et al.* 2008; Aveyard 2014: 18–20). These are, essentially, the destination and key landmarks for the journey of conducting the review and, if they are not clear and precise, you may well go off-track and fail to reach your intended destination.

The tasks of writing the question, aims and objectives for a review often sound as if they should be quite an easy part of the study. However, developing a clear and focused question, precise and achievable aims, and manageable objectives, all of which have clear links to, but do not repeat, one another, is often harder than it initially seems (Boren and Moxley 2015). In addition, although these elements can appear to be a very small part of the study as a whole, spending what may appear to be a disproportionate amount of time and effort in getting them right pays dividends. They are the foundation upon which the study as a whole rests.

Pitfall to avoid

Do not think that because they account for a relatively small number of words in your review the study question, aims and objectives are unimportant. The quality of the study as a whole depends on them, and they are worth spending time perfecting.

5.1 Why a clear, focused and answerable review question is important

In order to answer a question well, you need to know exactly what that question is, and precisely what it means. If your review question it not clear, it will be difficult for you to confidently design and conduct a study that will answer that question, or for your reader to know whether or not your review has addressed its question. That is not how you want to feel whilst you are carrying out your review, or how you want your reader to feel as they peruse the study report. If you have a clear question, your reader will know exactly what it is that you wanted to find out, and will therefore be able to assess whether or not you achieved this by the end of the study (Bragge 2010; Carman *et al.* 2013). Developing a clear and focused question is therefore a crucial part of any study, and merits considerable time and attention (Lipowski 2008).

Having a review question that is not clear and focused creates a very high chance that you will encounter difficulties in the rest of your study (Bragge 2010; Carman *et al.* 2013). If you consider your study as a journey to a particular piece of knowledge, having a destination that is vague or non-specific means that you will not know exactly where you are supposed to arrive at, which will make planning the journey rather difficult. You might travel in the right general direction for some time, but when you come to trying to find the precise location that you want, you will struggle, because you will not be clear about where that is. If, say, you arranged to meet a friend in 'Brighton' things might go well throughout both your journeys until you got to the outskirts of Brighton. However, finding each other would then be difficult without further clarification. It might, at that stage, become apparent that you were at opposite ends of the city, needed to negotiate a mutually convenient meeting place, navigate to it, and retrace some of the steps from your original journey. It would have been easier to have known all this to start with, and could have saved you some time and trouble. In the same way, having a precisely focused review question enables you to develop study methods that will enable you to get to exactly where you want to be (Borg Debono *et al.* 2013).

In the same way that recovering a journey that did not have a sufficiently precise destination can be corrected, it is possible to recover a study with a poor initial question by focusing more precisely at a later stage. However, this is often more difficult and time-consuming than developing a clear and focused question at the outset, and can mean that much of the effort that you have put in is wasted. If you are working to a tight schedule it may also make completing the review very difficult to achieve. For instance, as Chapter 6 describes, an early part of the literature review methodology process is to develop a strategy for searching the literature to find evidence related to your review question. This includes determining the keywords that you will search for in the literature. Having a clear and focused question enables you to develop the keywords required for your search with some confidence that they will address your question (Boren and Moxley 2015). On the other hand, having a question that is not clear, or not focused on what you really want to know about, means that the keywords you develop may not really reflect what you are interested in exploring. Having a clear and precise question should mean that your search can be designed to return a group of papers that are directly relevant to your study. Conversely, if it is vague, it is likely to mean that you find too much literature, much of which is not relevant to what you really want to know about. Whilst you may be able to wade through this, narrowing your focus as you go, the sheer volume of literature that you will have uncovered makes it very likely that you will pass over some potentially useful studies.

If, for example, you are exploring the evidence about short break care for people with severe learning disabilities, but are really interested in adults, your question must state this, and it should be included in your keywords. If not, your search will probably return a lot of information about children. This will mean that you gather evidence that is outside your main subject area, which may confuse the development of a clear evidence base as the issues for children may differ from those related to adults. In addition, because there will be considerably more literature for you to sort through, you may not be able to carry out as rigorous and systematic a selection process as you could with a narrower focus. This can lead to the inadvertent omission of important evidence or inclusion of irrelevant material.

Having a clear and focused review question should also enable you to stay on track as you progress your study. On your study journey, you will find plenty of diversions that you could take, and tempting asides.

If your question is clear, you are better placed to determine whether these will help you to get to your destination, or whether they will take you off-track, because you can constantly ask yourself: 'Does this contribute to answering my question?' However, if your review question is not clear and focused, there is a risk that you will be unsure as to whether some of the information that you find will contribute to answering it, or it will distract you. A well-thought-out study question therefore enables you to design and conduct a review that ensures that you answer it, and arrive at your intended destination, without being sidetracked by interesting, but irrelevant, distractions (Bragge 2010).

Pitfall to avoid

Avoid having a review question that is vaguely worded or too broad.

As well as being clear and focused, your review question needs to be answerable, and within the scope of the resources that are available to you, including time (Lipowski 2008; Offredy and Vickers 2010). If your initial question is: 'How adequate is the short break care offered to adults with severe learning disabilities?' that could, perhaps, be answered. However, the answer would need to include every permutation of what 'adequate' might mean, from the perspectives of various groups of people including: the person themselves, their family, professional carers, service organizers, etc. That would probably make it unanswerable in a single review, particularly if this was being undertaken as a relatively small, unfunded study. A review that is limited in breadth, but focused, rigorous and systematic, is much better than one that tries to answer every possible question within a broad subject area and, by so doing, answers no question adequately.

Pitfall to avoid

Do not think that the more you can cover in your review the better it will be. A tightly focused review that can be conducted rigorously and systematically is better than a broad, unwieldy review that lacks system and rigour.

Developing a clear, focused and answerable question is therefore a vital part of your review, and a necessary precursor to developing the aims, objectives and methods for the study.

5.2 Developing a focused review question

Your review question should usually only address one issue, because otherwise there is a risk that the study will become unwieldy and you will not achieve adequate rigour in any one area (Offredy and Vickers 2010). To draw an analogy with other types of question, it can be difficult if a person asks you a question that is really three or four questions. You may not know which one to answer first, answer each one rather superficially so as not to leave any part of the question unanswered, or get so involved in answering one of the questions that the others get forgotten. This is not what you want to happen in your literature review.

Deciding on the one thing that your review question will address often involves funnelling a broad question or area of interest down to something that is very clear, and precisely focused (Offredy and Vickers 2010). For example, if you work with people who have severe learning disabilities, and are interested in the provision of short break care for their families, you might decide to conduct a literature review about the quality of short break care for people with severe learning disabilities. This could appear to be a narrow enough area of practice, and amenable to one clearly focused question. It would indeed make a very good starting point, and narrows your focus down very well within the broad field of providing support for people with severe learning disabilities and their families. However, it would not provide you or your reader with a completely clear roadmap of exactly where you wanted to go within that area.

Within the area of short break care for people with severe learning disabilities, you would therefore need to more clearly delineate which particular group of people you were interested in: children, young adults, adults, older adults, etc. You would also need to consider which family members you were interested in: would this be the family members who provide day-to-day care for the person, a wider family group, or would you narrow it down to their parents (and if so what would you mean by the term 'parents')? Another consideration would be how you would define quality and from whose perspective this would be viewed.

You might feel that all of these permutations of the question are important areas, and they are. However, investigating them all in one review would be very likely to make it impossible to develop and maintain a clear focus throughout the study. You can always study other areas after completing your current review, and producing good quality evidence in a small, focused area is better than producing poor quality evidence that tries to cover too much. Your study, be it for academic purposes or not, will be judged on its quality in terms of answering the question posed, and being rigorous and systematic, not on how all-encompassing it attempted to be.

The process of developing a good study question therefore involves taking your initial topic and breaking each aspect of it down until you reach a decision about your exact focus. This can then be constructed into a question. Your question might, for instance, after some focusing, seem to be: 'How adequate is short break care for adults with severe learning disabilities?'. However, as you begin to consider this, you might ask yourself: 'What does adequate mean, and from whose perspective?' A clearer, more focused question might therefore be:

What are the views of the parents of adults with severe learning disabilities on the short break care that their child receives?

This makes it clear that the intended destination of your review journey is the views of parents of adults who have severe learning disabilities regarding the short break care that their child receives. The question could still be focused further, and the terms 'adult', 'parents' and 'short break care' will, as Chapter 4 identifies, need to be defined somewhere. However, this gives a fairly clear idea of your intended destination, and enables you to plan how to arrive there.

There are various tools or frameworks that can be employed to help you to focus your review question. No one of these is ideal for use in all circumstances, and you may find that you can focus your question without using such tools. However, they can be very useful in assisting you to determine exactly what it is that you want to explore, what the key components of your question will be, and to then frame your question around these (Bragge 2010; Guyatt et al. 2011).

5.3 Frameworks for developing your review question

5.3.1 The PICO framework

One well-established framework that can be used both for refining questions and developing strategies for searching the literature (as described in Chapter 6) is known as PICO (Cooke et al. 2012). PICO is a mnemonic for Population, Intervention, Comparison and Outcome, and, as this suggests, it requires the Population (P), Intervention (I), Comparison (C) and Outcome (O) that you plan to investigate to be detailed (Booth 2006; da Costa Santos *et al.* 2007; Bragge 2010; Guyatt *et al.* 2011). The PICO framework was designed primarily for questions that include interventions and comparisons, which makes it difficult to use in its original form for developing and refining questions that do not include these elements. However, other types of question may also be able to follow its principles (Bragge 2010; Guyatt *et al.* 2011). For example, the 'I' of intervention in the PICO mnemonic can be replaced by 'E' to represent exposure (Booth 2006). The PICO framework might, for instance, be used as follows to develop a review question regarding short break care for adults with severe learning disabilities:

P: The study population could be described as the parents of adults with severe learning disabilities.
I or E: In this example, the intervention or exposure would be short break care. This is perhaps not really an intervention, but it could be described as something that the population of interest is exposed to.
C: You might decide that your question will include a comparison, such as parents' views on two different approaches to short break care, perhaps short break care at home versus short break care outside the home. Equally, though, there might be no comparison made, and this part of the PICO framework could then be omitted. Remember that your study question does not need to be led by a tool. If making a comparison does not seem to fit the subject that you want to explore, or the way in which you wish to explore it, then you should not feel you need to include one simply so that you can use the PICO framework. The purpose of using a framework is to help you to develop a clear and focused question, not to create complications. Equally, whilst there may be no comparator in some questions, there may, in other situations, be multiple comparators (Guyatt *et al.* 2011). For instance, in this question, you might want to make comparisons between short break care at home, short break care in a residential setting, overnight short break care, day care, etc. Thinking through how many, if any, comparisons you want to make can also assist you to determine whether or not you will really be able to achieve all of this in your review. If you find that your comparisons are becoming numerous and complex, you may wish to reconsider whether or not this is an achievable goal within the time frame of your study. If it is not, then it gives you the chance to decide exactly what you think you will be able to achieve with the time and resources available to you, and what the most important comparisons are for the purpose of your review. You might, for instance, eventually decide that you will limit your intervention or exposure to short break care lasting

twenty-four hours or more, and then compare short break care of this duration in the person's home to short break care of this duration away from their home.

O: You may decide that you will focus on a particular outcome or outcomes, such as parents' degree of satisfaction with various forms of short break care. However, you may equally decide that the term 'outcome' will not really work for your review, because what you want to explore is parents' views, not outcomes per se.

As this chapter will go on to discuss, some questions, especially those that are likely to be drawing on qualitative evidence, do not easily fit the PICO framework. However, even if the PICO framework does not precisely fit your question, using its principles can help you to think about what you want to explore, even if you do not end up with a true PICO question. For example, using the process outlined above you could identify that the key concepts for your study will be:

- parents of adults with severe learning disabilities;
- short break care (of twenty-four hours' or more duration);
- a comparison between short break care at home and short break care outside the home;
- parents' views.

This could enable you to develop the question:

> What are the views of the parents of adults with severe learning disabilities on the short break care* that their child receives at home compared with the short break care that they receive outside their home? (*Short break care in this instance refers to care of twenty-four hours' or more duration.)

Pitfall to avoid

Do not try to make your question fit a particular tool or framework. Use a tool or framework to help you to develop your question.

The PICO framework is sometimes adapted to become the PICOT framework (Borg Debono et al. 2013; Carman et al. 2013). PICOT uses the same first four terms as PICO but adds the final letter 'T' (representing Time), to refer to the time frame for what will be studied (Riva et al. 2012; Borg Debono et al. 2013; Carman et al. 2013). For instance, using the PICOT framework the question about short break care for adults with severe learning disabilities might include 'short break care of more than twenty-four hours' duration' as the time frame.

The PICO and PICOT frameworks are widely used for developing questions and literature search strategies. However, their focus on interventions, comparisons and outcomes makes them most amenable to questions aimed at evaluating the evidence from quantitative, rather than qualitative, research (Cooke *et al.* 2012; Methley *et al.* 2014). There are other frameworks and tools that can more easily incorporate a wider range of study designs. The PICO framework has, for instance, been adapted by adding an 'S' (making it the PICOS framework), wherein the 'S' refers to the study design (Methley *et al.* 2014). This allows for clarification of the type of evidence that is of interest. In the example concerning short break care for adults with severe learning disabilities, the PICOS framework might produce something like:

P: The parents of adults with severe learning disabilities;
I (E): Short break care (of twenty-four hours' or more duration);
C: Short break care at home compared to short break away from the home;
O: No outcome stated;
S: Qualitative research, related to parents' views.

This would enable a question to be developed that stated:

> What is the evidence from qualitative research concerning the views of the parents of adults with severe learning disabilities on the short break care that their child receives at home compared with the short break care* that they receive outside their home? (*Short break care in this instance refers to care of twenty-four hours' or more duration.)

Nevertheless, even with this adaptation, the rather quantitative focus of the ingredients of the rest of the PICOS mnemonic remains. Consequently, some tools have been developed specifically to assist in designing questions and search strategies for reviews that may include qualitative research, quantitative research, or a mix of both types of evidence. One such tool is the SPICE framework (Booth 2004, 2006; Cooke *et al.* 2012).

5.3.2 The SPICE framework

The SPICE framework requires the following study elements to be identified:

S: the Setting. This might be the location of interest, or the particular characteristics of the setting that are of interest. In the example concerning short break care for adults with severe learning disabilities, it could be England, or it could be situations in which adults with severe learning disabilities are cared for at home, by their parent(s).

P: the Perspective. This refers to the perspective being explored: in the example in question, the views of parents of adults with severe learning disabilities would be the perspective of interest.

I: the Intervention. As with the PICO framework, this refers to the intervention or exposure that is being investigated. This would, therefore, again be short break care lasting twenty-four hours or more.

C: the Comparison. Like the PICO framework, this refers to what, if anything, will be compared in the study. In this instance, it might again be short break care at the person's home compared to short break care outside their home.

E: the Evaluation. The evaluation element of the SPICE framework refers to the manner in which the studies in the review are expected to have evaluated the intervention of interest. The SPICE framework uses the term 'evaluation' rather than 'outcome' because it means that the issue can be evaluated using something other than measurable outcomes. In the example in question, the comparison between care at home versus care outside the home environment would be evaluated using parents' views of each type of service.

The SPICE mnemonic could therefore be used to develop the question:

> What are the views of parents of adults with severe learning disabilities who are cared for at home on the short break care* that their child receives at home, compared with the short break care that they receive outside their home? (*Short break care refers to care of twenty-four hours' or more duration.)

However, despite providing for a broader range of review questions than the PICO framework, the SPICE framework is not universally considered to cater well for studies aimed at generating or reviewing qualitative research (Cooke et al. 2012). An alternative tool, which has been designed specifically for the development of questions or searches related to qualitative evidence, is the *SPIDER* framework (Cooke et al. 2012).

5.3.3 The *SPIDER* framework

The *SPIDER* mnemonic works as follows:

S: the Sample. Because the findings from qualitative research are not usually intended to be generalizable in the way that quantitative findings aim to be, the term 'sample' rather than 'population' is used in the *SPIDER* framework. This term indicates that the focus is on those who participated in the research, not a population to which generalization is intended (Cooke *et al.* 2012). In the example that has been used previously in this chapter, the sample would be the parents of adults who have severe learning disabilities.

PI: the Phenomenon of Interest. Because the aim of qualitative research is often to understand behaviours, decisions and individual experiences the term 'phenomenon of interest' is used in the *SPIDER* framework rather than terms such as 'intervention' or 'exposure'. In the example in question, the phenomenon of interest would be short break care (of more than twenty-four hours' duration) for adults with severe learning disabilities.

D: the Design. This refers to the design of the study or studies, and forms a part of the *SPIDER* framework because the study design influences the type of information that is likely to be obtained. It is a particularly valuable part of the framework when it is being used to develop searches. However, it can also be useful in designing study questions when it will be helpful to include the type of evidence that is to be incorporated into the question.

E: the Evaluation. In the *SPIDER* framework the term 'evaluation' is used rather than 'outcome' as the findings from qualitative research are not usually reported in terms of outcomes. In the example that has been used previously in this chapter, the views of parents of adults with severe learning disabilities would be the means of evaluation.

R: the Research type. This element of the *SPIDER* framework, like study design, enables the tool to be used to determine the type of evidence that will be required or used (Cooke *et al.* 2012, Methley *et al.* 2014). This is especially useful in making decisions about what terms will be included in the search for relevant literature, as described in Chapter 6. In addition, like the study design, it can also be useful for clarifying what type of evidence will be drawn on in a literature review.

The *SPIDER* framework would, therefore, enable the development of a question such as:

What is the evidence from qualitative research on the views of parents of adults with severe learning disabilities regarding the short break care (of twenty-four hours' or more duration) that their child receives?

However, whilst these frameworks or tools can be useful, they will only enhance the development of a study question if they are used appropriately. Trying to force a topic area to fit into an inappropriate framework will not be helpful, and it is therefore worth considering whether a particular tool matches the subject that you want to investigate. Notwithstanding their value, solely using a tool will not enable you to design a good question. What is required is for you to think, carefully, about exactly what you want to study, and precisely what you mean by each of the things that you think you want to study.

> ## Pitfall to avoid
>
> Do not rely on a framework or tool to develop your study question for you: use it to help you to develop your thinking about your study question.

Having identified your review question, the next step of the process is to develop the aims of your review.

5.4 Developing the aims of the review

In addition to the question that the review seeks to answer, most studies that use literature review methodology should have aims. Having a clear review question means that you know precisely what you want to find out, whereas the aims of a review clarify exactly what you hope to achieve in order to answer that question (Denscombe 2012).

Because the aims of your review should indicate what you intend to accomplish in order to address your review question, they should not go beyond the scope of your question. They should also be realistic and achievable (Denscombe 2012). As you develop them, you should ask yourself:

Will this help to answer my study question?
Could I achieve all of this in one study?
Can I achieve this in the time, and with the resources, that I have?

If the answer to any of these questions is 'no', or 'unlikely', you should reconsider your aims, and see if they have drifted beyond the scope of the study question. If your aims have gone beyond the remit of your review question, then you should revise them, being guided by the study question, and ensuring that your aims address that, and that alone. If your aims are very tightly associated with the review question, but seem unachievable, you probably need to revisit your question as well as your aims.

Your aims therefore need to stay very close to the review question. They should not be a repetition of it, but should be directly linked to it. If your aims drift away from the question, then as you design and conduct the review you risk either following the aims and not answering the question, or answering the question and not meeting the aims of the review. At best, you will give yourself additional, and confusing, work, trying to effectively conduct two studies: one addressing the review aims and one answering the review question. If your question and aims are not a logical continuation of one another, not only will you struggle, but your reader will have difficulty in following what is being done and why it is being done.

As Chapter 3 outlined, the quality of a study is largely judged on whether it is rigorous and systematic. If meeting the aims of a study would clearly result in the study question being answered, then this suggests that there is system in that part of the study design. If, on the other hand, achieving the study aims would not answer the study question, then system is lacking. Therefore, as you develop the aims for your review it is useful to constantly cross-check to ensure that each of your stated aims will contribute to answering your review question.

For example, if you have decided that your review question will be:

> What are the views of parents of adults with severe learning disabilities on the short break care that their child receives at home compared to the short break care that they receive away from home?

your aims all need to be directly related to this. They might be:

- to identify the views of parents of adults with severe learning disabilities on the short break care that their child receives at home;
- to identify the views of parents of adults with severe learning disabilities on the short break care that their child receives outside the home environment;

- to compare the views of parents of adults with severe learning disabilities on the short break care that their child receives at home to that provided outside the home environment.

If you succeeded in meeting these aims, you should be able to answer the review question, and not be taken off-track. If, on the other hand, you developed an aim that said something like: 'To explore the effect of short break care on parents' relationships' it would move your review towards evaluating the evidence on the effects of short break care, or the effects of having a child with severe learning disabilities, on parents' relationships. Exploring parents' views may, of course, unearth their views on how short break care affects their relationships, but ascertaining that particular piece of information would not be a specific aim of the review. It might become a finding: for example that parents are of the opinion that out of home short break care gives them time together which enhances their relationships. Nonetheless, as an aim, it would suggest a different question, such as 'What influence does short break care have on the relationships of parents of adults who have severe learning disabilities?'.

As you consider the aims of your review, you may find it useful to revisit any framework or tool that you used to develop the study question. This enables you to ensure that the key issues identified by using that framework are the main points addressed in both the review question and the aims. In addition, it allows you to check whether or not you included a comparison in the study question. If you did, you should ensure that your aims also include a comparison. If, on the other hand, the tool you used and your question have not included a comparison, your aims should not. Box 5.1 shows how a study's aims could be matched against the elements of the SPICE framework.

Pitfall to avoid

Do not feel that your aims need to cover more than your review question does. They should enable you to answer your question, but should not go beyond it.

Developing and reviewing your aims also provides you with a useful opportunity to check that your study is not biased. The fact that you have chosen a particular subject to study means that you are probably interested in it, and have experience and views about it. However, you need to ensure that your review gains an impartial answer to the study question. For instance, if your question is:

Box 5.1

Study aims related to the SPICE framework

SPICE framework:

S: The situation in which adults with severe learning disabilities are being cared for at home by their parent(s).
P: The perspectives of the parents of adults with severe learning disabilities.
I: Short break care of more than twenty-four hours' duration.
C: Short break care at the person's home compared to short break care outside their home.
E: Parents' views.

Study aims:

• To identify the views of parents of adults with severe learning disabilities on the short break care that their child receives at home: would cover the concepts S, P, I, E.
• To identify the views of parents of adults with severe learning disabilities on the short break care that their child receives outside the home environment: would cover the concepts S, P, I, E.
• To compare the views of parents of adults with severe learning disabilities on the short break care that their child receives at home to that provided outside the home environment: would cover the concept C.

What are the views of parents of adults with severe learning disabilities on the short break care* that their child receives at home compared with the short break care that they receive outside their home? (*Short break care refers to care of twenty-four hours' or more duration.)

the answer has to be able to include all views, positive, negative and neutral, about both types of short break care. It also has to be possible to obtain answers that you did not expect, or which run contrary to your own views. If one of your aims was: 'To identify the ways in which short break care assists parents of adults with severe learning disabilities to remain in employment' you might be demonstrating that your view is that short break care helps parents to remain in employment. However, this might not be how parents perceive short break care. A more neutral aim might be: 'To ascertain whether short break care influences employment opportunities for parents of adults with severe learning disabilities'. Reviewing the exact wording of your aims, and considering whether there is any suggestion of bias, can assist you to identify whether there is a risk of your existing views influencing the review, as well as whether your aims really address the review question.

| Pitfall to avoid |

Do not be tempted to think that the more aims you have the better your review will be. A concise, achievable list of relevant aims is best.

The aims of your review tell you what the study needs to achieve. It can be tempting to think that, in order to produce a good quality review, you need a lot of aims. However, a short, but specific, achievable and relevant list of aims is much better than a long, unwieldy list that detracts from the focus of the study. Like the review question, the aims are worth spending some time on developing. Once your aims have been established, the next task is to formulate the objectives of the review.

5.5 Review objectives: what they are and how to develop them

The aims of your review refer to what you hope to achieve in the study, whereas the objectives describe the steps that you will take to ensure that you meet your aims. The review question, aims and objectives should therefore work logically together: meeting the aims will enable the review question to be answered, and fulfilling the objectives will enable the aims to be achieved. For a study to be considered systematic, the question, aims and objectives should therefore all be a logical continuation of one another (Lipowski 2008; Offredy and Vickers 2010).

Because the objectives of the review should relate to actions that will be taken to achieve the study aims, they are usually stated using words that imply action (Offredy and Vickers 2010). In addition, like the review question and aims, they should be clear, and each objective should, ideally, concern only one action (Offredy and Vickers 2010). This makes it easier for you and your reader to identify these individual actions, and to match them against the aims of the review. If an objective is composed of more than one action, it makes it more difficult to see which aim or aims it assists in meeting. Having more than one action in each statement also increases the chance of irrelevant objectives creeping in, or of you ending up trying to fulfil too many objectives.

Pitfall to avoid

Do not include objectives that will not contribute to meeting any of the aims of your review.

Whether or not your objectives have been met will give you, and those who read your study, an indication of whether or not the review has been successful. Your objectives should, therefore, describe things that can be noted as being as completed or not (Kumar 2005). In this sense, they should be observable (Offredy and Vickers 2010). Whether the objectives of the review have been accomplished or not will be a criterion against which your study's success will be measured: your objectives should, therefore, also be achievable (Offredy and Vickers 2010). Because the study objectives should describe actions that will enable you to achieve your study aims, if you have not fulfilled them it suggests that either:

you have not met your aims (and, by implication, not answered your question)

or

there has not been a systematic and rigorous approach to developing the study question, aims and objectives, because some of these have been achieved independently of the others.

As with the development of the study aims, if you look at your objectives and feel they will not be achievable, then you need to review them, and consider whether they are all required in order to meet the aims of the review. If they are not, then you should revisit them, ensuring that you are only attempting to carry out actions that will address the study aims. If they are all required in order to meet your aims, but are unachievable, then the review's aims (and, as described in the previous section, perhaps the review question) also need to be reviewed.

For example, for the question and aims:

What are the views of parents of adults with severe learning disabilities on the short break care* that their child receives at home compared to the short break care that they receive outside of the home? (*Defined as care of twenty-four hours' or more duration.)

your aims all need to relate to this. They might, as detailed above, be:

1 to identify the views of parents of adults with severe learning disabilities on the short break care that their child receives at home;
2 to identify the views of parents of adults with severe learning disabilities on the short break care that their child receives outside the home environment;
3 to compare the views of parents of adults with severe learning disabilities on the short break care that their child receives at home to that provided outside the home environment.

The objectives could then be:

1 to evaluate the existing published research regarding the views of parents of adults with severe learning disabilities on short break care provided outside the home environment;
2 to synthesize the evidence derived from objective 1 in order to ascertain the current evidence on the views of parents of adults with severe learning disabilities regarding short break care outside the home environment;
3 to evaluate the existing published research regarding the views of parents of adults with severe learning disabilities on short break care provided at home;
4 to synthesize this evidence derived from objective 3 in order to ascertain the current evidence on the views of parents of adults with severe learning disabilities regarding short break care provided at home;
5 to use the evidence derived from objectives 2 and 4 to compare the views of parents of adults with severe learning disabilities regarding short break care provided at home and short break care provided outside the home environment.

By doing these five things, or meeting these objectives, the aims of the study should be met, and the review question answered. In addition, they do not go outside the remit of the review question or aims. They describe actions that, if taken, will address the study aims. In this way they are similar, and clearly linked to, but do not repeat, the aims of the review.

It can be tempting to confuse the review objectives with the review methods, because both concern the steps that are taken in order to achieve the study aim and answer the study question. However, as Chapters 6, 7 and 8 describe, the review methods detail the exact steps that are taken to conduct the review. The objectives do not need to enter into the detail that the methods do of every stage of the process of conducting the review: they are a broader statement of what will, in principle, be done in order to achieve the study aims. They may, for instance, state that evidence from published research will be evaluated. The details of how this was achieved would, however, be provided in the methods section of the review. In the same way that the review question leads to the aims, which lead to the objectives, the objectives should, therefore, logically lead to the study methods.

Summary

Having a clear review question, aims and objectives enable your study to be focused, and ensuring that the three are logically and clearly related to each other are important steps towards your review being rigorous and systematic. Your review question, aims and objectives should be achievable within the time and resources available to you, and generally a tightly focused question will result in a better quality study than one that seeks to cover too much ground. In addition, if the question, aims and objectives of your study are clear, it will assist in developing systematic and rigorous methods for your review, because what you want to achieve and how you intend to achieve it will be evident.

Terminology

Aims: the aims of a review should detail what you intend to achieve by undertaking the study.

Objectives: the objectives of a review should state the actions that you intend to take to enable you to achieve the study aims.

PICO: a mnemonic designed to assist in developing study questions and search strategies. The PICO framework requires the Population (P), Intervention (I), Comparison (C) and Outcome (O) of interest in to be detailed.

SPICE: a mnemonic designed to assist in developing study questions and search strategies. The SPICE mnemonic represents: S: Setting, P: Perspective, I: Intervention, C: Comparison, E: Evaluation.

SPIDER: a mnemonic designed to assist in developing study questions and search strategies, especially those concerned with qualitative research. The *SPIDER* mnemonic represents: S: Sample, PI: Phenomenon of Interest, D: Design, E: Evaluation, R: Research type.

Chapter 6
Carrying out the search

Key points:

- The process of searching for literature should be systematic, rigorous and focused on the review question.
- Searching effectively for literature to include in a review involves: formulating key concepts; determining keywords and their synonyms; deciding where to search; and developing inclusion and exclusion criteria.
- The decisions made at each stage of the search should be carefully considered so as to ensure that the review is rigorous and systematic, but also manageable.
- A careful record should be kept of the decisions made and the literature that is retrieved.

Having identified the question, aims and objectives for your review, the next stage in the process of conducting a study that uses literature review methodology is to gather the data that will enable you to address these. This is achieved by searching the existing literature.

The data collection process in any type of research should be systematic, rigorous, unbiased and designed to ensure that the study question is answered. The same applies to the process of gathering data for a study that uses literature review methodology. How the first step in the process of gathering data, the search for literature, is conducted is therefore a crucial contribution to the quality of the study (Kamienski *et al.* 2013). In order to be as certain as possible that you retrieve all the relevant literature, a systematic and rigorous approach to designing and conducting the search is required (Aveyard 2014: 74). If this is not achieved, then the study will not be able to claim to present the current best evidence, because some of that evidence may be missing. Your strategy for searching the literature therefore needs to enable you to find all the literature that is relevant to your question, and the minimum possible amount of irrelevant information (Waltho *et al.* 2015). You also need to present this in a way that details clearly for your reader how the evidence presented in the review was sought (Hemingway and Brereton 2009; Murphy *et al.* 2009; Bettany-Saltikov 2010). This chapter outlines steps and strategies that will assist you in achieving this.

6.1 Formulation of key concepts

6.1.1 Keywords

The first step towards successfully searching for something is to decide exactly what it is that you want to find (and what you do not want to find). Searching for literature is no different, and the start point for devising your search strategy is therefore to develop a description of precisely what you are looking for. Generally, this description is then fed into some kind of electronic processing system, which looks for what you said you wanted and produces a list of results for you to peruse. Because you feed the description into a machine, it needs to be clear, and stated in a language that the machine understands. The first part of developing this description is to decide on the terms that you want to look for. These need to be stated accurately, because the words that you ask for are exactly what the machine will look for.

> ### Pitfall to avoid
>
> Do not assume that an electronic search facility will consider whether what you have asked it to search for makes sense. It will usually just search for exactly what you requested.

Many electronic search facilities ask you to enter keywords or phrases of interest, and then browse through vast amounts of information searching for these terms (Levy and Ellis 2006). You are then presented with a list of everything that has been found that contains the words or phrases that you asked for. So whilst you will, as Chapter 5 discusses, have spent some time in developing a question that describes exactly what you want to look for, you will need to reduce that question back to keywords or phrases in order to enter it into a search facility. If you enter the whole question, the search facility may think that it has been instructed to find everything with any of those words in it, many of which will not be related to what you really want to know about (Poojary and Bagadia 2014). For example, if your review question was:

> Is using a recorded handover as effective as using a face-to-face handover for nurses on acute wards?

putting that question into an electronic search facility that utilizes keywords or phrases could mean that your results included every document that had the word 'using' in it. At best, that would waste an awful lot of your time. In terms of study quality, it would be very likely to mean that you were unable to give as much attention as you should to filtering the relevant articles from all those that were found, as the volume would be way too high for you to achieve this.

As Chapter 5 identifies, your study question will be built around certain key concepts that also form the basis for the study aims and objectives. These are the words or phrases that you need to focus on as you develop your search strategy. If, as described in Chapter 5, you used a framework such as PICO, *SPIDER* or SPICE to develop your study question, the terms listed against each letter of the mnemonic are your key concepts. For the question:

> Is using a recorded handover as effective as using a face-to-face handover for nurses on acute wards?

you might have used PICO to develop the terms:

> Population: nurses on acute wards;
> Intervention: handover;
> Comparison: recorded or face-to-face;
> Outcome: effectiveness (you would, in the background, rationale or process of developing your study question, need to state how you have defined 'effectiveness' in this context).

Your key concepts, taken from your PICO framework, could then be:

> acute wards;
> nurses;
> handover;
> face-to-face;
> recorded;
> effectiveness.

However, not all of these terms would necessarily be things you wanted to include in your search. If this was your question, your main interest would probably be in searching for information on recorded nursing handovers, so you would be interested in an article called: 'The effectiveness of recorded nursing handovers' but probably not an article entitled 'The effectiveness of nursing handovers'. In addition, although your review question requires you to make a judgement about the effectiveness of recorded versus face-to-face nursing hand-overs, not all the documents that are relevant to your review may have the word 'effectiveness' in them. An article entitled: 'Nurses' experiences of introducing recorded handovers' might well be relevant to your review, even though it does not specify that the study aimed to determine the effectiveness of different types of handover. Your keywords or terms for the purpose of searching the literature might, therefore, actually be:

> acute wards;
> recorded;
> nurses' handover.

Pitfall to avoid

Avoid entering terms into your search that do not reflect the key points that you want to consider. Anything that you enter will be searched for.

Using only these three key terms in your search would, nonetheless, probably not unearth all the relevant evidence about your question: you would also need to consider words that had the same meaning as these terms.

6.1.2 Synonyms

There are often words or terms that could be used interchangeably with each of the keywords that you develop for your search. As well as defining your key terms, you therefore also need to identify other words or phrases that could be considered synonymous with these, and include them in your search (Holland 2007; Cronin et al. 2008; Aveyard 2014: 82–4). For instance, 'acute wards' might also be described in the literature as: 'inpatient', 'wards', 'medical wards' or 'surgical wards'. These words or terms are not all strictly synonymous with the term 'acute wards' ('inpatient wards' could, for example, include long stay or rehabilitation wards, as well as acute wards). However, someone writing an article about the use of recorded hand-overs on acute wards might use the title: 'A comparison of recorded and face-to-face nursing handovers on inpatient wards'. You would probably want to access this article, even though the terms 'inpatient' and 'acute ward' are not entirely synonymous in other contexts. Therefore, when you identify synonyms for your search, you need to think not just about whether the words that you select are precisely synonymous, but whether they have the potential to be used as contextually synonymous in literature about the subject in question.

In your quest to unearth the full range of synonyms, as well as thinking of current terminology, you should consider how terms may have changed over time (Levy and Ellis 2006). For example, if your question is:

> Is using a recorded handover as effective as using a face-to-face handover for nurses on acute wards?

the term 'handover' might historically have been referred to as 'report'. In addition, whilst the term 'recorded' is useful because it covers all recording devices, the term 'taped' might previously have been used to refer to recording handovers using a tape recorder. As this chapter will go on to discuss, you may decide to limit the time span of the literature that you gather, and historic considerations may be less relevant if you decide to limit your search to literature from within the past five years. The decisions you make about the synonyms you use in your search need to be clear, consistent with other decisions that you make, and justified.

You may have a very good idea of what the synonyms for your keywords are. However, as well as using all the terms that you can think of, you need to take steps to systematically and rigorously ensure that you have identified all of the possible synonyms. To achieve this, you can use a thesaurus, and also check the articles you begin to retrieve to see if they contain any synonyms that you have omitted (Levy and Ellis 2006). If they do, you should rerun any searches necessary with the newly identified synonyms included.

6.1.3 Abbreviations and spelling variations

Because an electronic search will uncover, letter for letter, exactly what you ask it to, as well as identifying words that might be used interchangeably, you should consider whether there are any spelling variations in your keywords and their synonyms. For instance, the British English term 'paediatric' and the American English term 'pediatric' would not both be found by a search in which you entered the word 'paediatric'. Any abbreviations or acronyms that might be used to represent your keywords should also be identified. If, for example, your review concerned the accident and emergency department, you should include abbreviations such as A&E in your search as this might be the term used in documents on the subject. If your key terms include any medications, both the generic and commonly used brand names for these should be identified in your search strategy (Thames Valley Literature Review Standards Group 2006; Holland 2007).

> ### Pitfall to avoid
>
> Do not skimp on the time taken to carefully identify your keywords and their synonyms. This is a part of your data collection strategy, and if it is poorly performed your data collection process will not be systematic and rigorous.

Table 6.1 shows some alternative terms that could be used for the keywords and phrases in the question: 'Is using a recorded handover as effective as using a face-to-face handover for nurses on acute wards?' Making a list or table of this type can help you to be sure that you have identified all your keywords and their alternatives, and enables you to check that you include them all in your search. It also demonstrates to your reader the rigour of the process that you used (Murphy et al. 2009).

The terms that you have identified, including synonyms and different spellings, should all be included in your search. However, if they are all entered into an electronic search together, they will produce a lot of irrelevant material, as the search facility will look for documents with any of these words in the section that you have asked it to search in. It would, for instance, produce every document that it found with the term 'medical ward' in the title or abstract, regardless of whether the article contained any information about nursing handovers. Having identified these terms, the next step is therefore to use them in a way that means that you get all the information that you need, but as little as possible irrelevant material. One approach to achieving this is to use Boolean operators.

Table 6.1 Examples of search terms

Keyword	Synonym 1	Synonym 2	Synonym 3	Synonym 4	Synonym 5
nursing handover	nursing report	nurses' handover	nurses' report		
recorded	taped	record	tape	recording	taping
acute ward	inpatient	medical ward	surgical ward	ward	

6.1.4 Boolean operators

In the context of searching the literature, the terms 'and', 'or' and 'not' are often referred to as Boolean terms or the use of Boolean logic (named after George Boole, who devised this system). Using these words in the right way can make your search for information more focused and precise, and save you from spending a lot of time looking through irrelevant information (providing the database that you use supports them). Using Boolean logic enables you to instruct the search facility you are using not just about what words you want to find, but also what combinations of words you are interested in finding (Holland 2007).

1   **And**

Using the Boolean operator 'and' instructs your search facility to only extract documents that contain all of the terms linked by the 'and' command (Kamienski *et al.* 2013; Waltho *et al.* 2015). For example, if you were comparing recorded handovers with non-recorded handovers, you would not want all the documents in any given database that mentioned the word 'handover'. You would only want articles that included the term 'handover' and the concept of this being recorded. By entering 'handover AND recorded' in your search, you would exclude documents that had the words 'handover' or 'recorded' but not both of these terms in them. Using this approach, you would get an article entitled: 'How effective is a recorded nursing handover?' but not 'What are relatives' views on nursing handovers?' The Boolean 'and' operator therefore assists in focusing the search on your question.

2   **Or**

The Boolean term 'or' is used to identify terms that will be accepted as interchangeable for the purposes of your search, such as your synonyms (Kamienski *et al.* 2013; Waltho *et al.* 2015). Using it means that you do not have to carry out a separate search for each synonym, because you can indicate to the electronic search facility you are using that certain words have been deemed to mean the same.

You can also use more than one Boolean operator in a search. For instance, by using the Boolean 'or' operator alongside the 'and' operator you could search for: 'recorded OR taped AND handover' at the same time. This would enable the search to locate all the records that contained the word 'handover' and the word 'recorded' followed by all the records that contained the word 'handover' and the word 'taped' and then combine both groups of records into a single set. So although two searches were performed, you would only have to set up one search and would be presented with one list of all the retrieved documents that contained either of the two keywords 'recorded' and 'taped' alongside the keyword 'handover'.

3 **Not**

The Boolean term 'not' can be used to narrow your search by making sure that any document that contains a particular term is excluded from the results (Holland 2007; Kamienski *et al.* 2013; Waltho *et al.* 2015). If you want to search for information about recorded nursing handovers on acute wards but do not want to receive any articles about handovers on acute psychiatric wards, you could search for: 'handover AND acute NOT psychiatric'. This would mean that any documents that refer to psychiatric wards would be excluded from your search results.

The 'not' operator can be very valuable for excluding irrelevant information, but you should be aware that its exclusion of words is absolute and overrides any conflicting inclusions (Aveyard 2014: 85–6). So, if you searched for: 'handover AND acute NOT psychiatric' the search would exclude an article entitled 'Recorded nursing handovers in acute medical and acute psychiatric wards' because the 'not' outweighs the other words, even though at least one part of that document might be useful to you.

Many search facilities support the use of Boolean logic, whilst others use their own system to achieve the same effect as Boolean terms do. This often appears in the 'advanced search' option, and it is sensible to check whether your search facility supports the use of Boolean logic or uses an equivalent system. If you try to use Boolean operators in a system that does not support them the 'and', 'or' and 'not' commands will not work, and you may find that you have inadvertently searched for every document that contains any of the words 'and', 'or' or 'not'.

Pitfall to avoid

Check if and how the search facility you are using supports Boolean logic or a similar system before running your search.

6.1.5 Truncation and wildcards

Boolean logic's 'and', 'or' and 'not' functions enable you to search efficiently using the keywords or phrases that you have developed, and their synonyms. However, you will often need to include variations of the same root word in your search. For instance, if you want to search for information about recorded nursing handovers, as shown in Table 6.1, the root word 'record' could also appear as 'recording' or 'recorded' in article titles, keywords or abstracts. Typing in three searches to account for this, or adding a Boolean 'or' for every permutation of every word, would be very time-consuming. Fortunately, because these words all share the common stem 'record', a process called truncation can be used to enable you to use the shortest version of the word, with a truncation character (usually a *) to represent a range of possible endings (Holland 2007; Waltho et al. 2015). In this case, you could use record* to represent record, recorded and recording.

If any of the words that you want to search for have slightly different spelling options within them, you can use a wildcard character instead of the truncation process to capture these. The wildcard character (usually a * or a ?) instructs the search tool to look for any (or no) letter in that space (Holland 2007; Waltho et al. 2015). Using the wildcard function, anaesthetic could be searched for as an*esthetic to capture both the North American and British spellings.

Using Boolean operators, truncation and wildcards, a search strategy for literature related to the question:

Is using a recorded handover as effective as using a face-to-face handover for nurses on acute wards?

could be something like that shown in Box 6.1.

Box 6.1

Search strategy for the question: 'Is using a recorded handover as effective as using a face-to-face handover for nurses on acute wards?'

Search 1: Nurs* handover AND record* OR tap* AND acute ward*
Search 2: Nurs* report AND record* OR tap* AND acute ward*
Search 3: Nurs* handover AND record* OR tap* AND medical ward*
Search 4: Nurs* report AND record* OR tap* AND medical ward*
Search 5: Nurs* handover AND record* OR tap* AND surgical ward*
Search 6: Nurs* report AND record* OR tap* AND surgical ward*
Search 7: Nurs* handover AND record* OR tap* AND inpatient
Search 8: Nurs* report AND record* OR tap* AND inpatient
Search 9: Nurs* handover AND record* OR tap* AND ward*
Search 10: Nurs* report AND record* OR tap* AND ward*

6.2 Searching in the right field

When you search an electronic database, you can usually choose where in a document you want to look for the words that you are interested in finding (also referred to as which field you want to search in). The options offered generally include the documents' author, keywords, title, title and abstract, or the whole document (Levy and Ellis 2006). If you select the wrong field, you are unlikely to get the information you need. For example, if you are searching for 'nurs*' (to represent nurse, nurses and nursing) and select to search in the journal title field you will get all the articles in every journal that has the word nurse, nursing or nurses in its title, which would be very unhelpful.

If you are carrying out a keyword search, you will usually be best advised to search within the document abstracts, titles and keywords (Aveyard 2014: 86). Occasionally it may be appropriate to search in the whole article, however this can produce rather a wide range of documents as it effectively retrieves every piece of literature encountered that has the stated keywords anywhere in it. This is likely to include a lot of irrelevant documents. If you were looking for information about recorded nursing handovers and searched for: 'nurs* AND record* AND handover' in the whole article you would retrieve any document that had these three words anywhere in it, even if they were not linked with each other and not the focus of the article.

Although you will therefore usually be best advised to search in the keywords, abstract and title fields, searching other fields can also be useful. If, for instance, you have identified a particular author who has written a great deal on a subject you can search for their name in the author field in order to check that you have not missed any of their work.

Having identified your keywords and synonyms, decided how these should be arranged in your search and where in the document you want to search for them, you should be fairly confident of accessing the vast majority of relevant articles and not too many irrelevant ones. However, there are some further steps to take to ensure that your review includes all the relevant evidence, and the minimum possible amount of irrelevant information. Some of these steps can be included in your search, but even the most focused search will often return some documents that fall outside the remit of your question. As you read the titles, abstracts and whole texts of the articles that you retrieve, you may therefore still decide to discard some. To make sure that this process is conducted systematically, rigorously and without bias, you should develop exclusion and inclusion criteria that will guide your decision-making (Cronin *et al.* 2008; Aveyard 2014: 74–80).

6.3 Developing inclusion and exclusion criteria

The inclusion and exclusion criteria for your study are the rules that set out what attributes the documents that are included in the final review should or should not have. Developing clear inclusion and exclusion criteria will mean that it is clear to you, and your reader, why each of the documents included in the review was deemed to be suitable and why those that were excluded were not. It will also enable you to demonstrate that these decisions were based on a logical, systematic and unbiased process.

Often, the inclusion criteria are the direct opposite of the exclusion criteria. One very commonly used criterion pertains to the type of literature that will be included in the review. If one of the inclusion criteria is that only primary research will be used, then the corresponding exclusion criteria would be any documents that do not report on primary research. However, not every inclusion criterion will necessarily have such a direct opposite exclusion criterion.

6.3.1 The type of literature that will be included in the review

As identified above, the type of literature that you are interested in is usually one of the criteria for inclusion or exclusion in a review. Your decision about what types of literature you will include will be guided by several factors, including the nature of your question, and the type of evidence that exists or is likely to exist on the subject. Your goal is to carry out a complete, but highly focused, review, and your background reading and the subject matter will probably have given you a good indication of what would be a reasoned and reasonable decision here. In some cases you may decide that you can and should review all evidence of all types. However, in other instances, selecting only one type of evidence will be appropriate, to enable you to make more precise comparisons, and conduct a manageable study. How you make the decision as to which type or types of evidence you will use in your review may be guided by considering hierarchies of evidence.

Hierarchies of evidence were developed to indicate which forms of evidence are considered, in principle, to be the best. Such hierarchies typically grade the worth of evidence according to how well it can be generalized. The pinnacle of evidence in such hierarchies is therefore usually Systematic Reviews that use meta-analysis (which are discussed in Chapter 7), followed by Randomized Controlled Trials.

Other forms of quantitative research are placed further down in the hierarchy, followed by non-research-based sources of evidence such as case reports and expert opinion (Roecker 2012). The place of qualitative research in such hierarchies presents a challenge because its intention is not to produce generalizable results. Therefore, despite its importance, meaningfully incorporating it into a system in which generalizability is the key quality indicator is problematic. Another difficulty with relying on hierarchies of evidence is that they deal with the type, not necessarily the quality, of the evidence in question (for example, a low-quality randomized controlled trial would be graded more highly than a very diligently performed case control study) (Burns *et al.* 2011).

One of the advantages of such hierarchies of evidence is, nevertheless, that they demonstrate that some forms of evidence are, in principle, more worthy of trust than others. However, consideration must still be given to what any particular piece of evidence is for, and that generalizability is not the key quality indicator in all situations should be recognized (Glasziou *et al.* 2004). For example, it might be shown almost unequivocally from the evidence derived from a quantitative experiment that listening to a recorded nursing handover is as effective as attending a face-to-face handover in terms of conveying information. However, it might be equally essential to have an understanding, derived from qualitative data or case reports, concerning whether nursing staff find this approach user-friendly, and why they would, or would not, use it.

Therefore, whilst such hierarchies have a place in guiding your thinking about the types of evidence that you will include in your review, your decision should be based on how appropriate particular types of evidence are for addressing your review question. You will also need to consider the practicalities of how manageable your review will be. For instance, you may expect to uncover a lot of evidence on the subject of recorded nursing handovers and have limited time and resources with which to conduct your review. In this situation you could decide that, as hierarchies of evidence place research as a higher form of evidence than expert opinion or case reports, you will only include documents that report on research in your review. However, because the subject may be equally amenable to investigation using qualitative, quantitative or mixed methods research, you might decide that you will use any of these types of research.

You will also need to determine whether you will include both the published and unpublished (or 'grey') literature in your review (Cronin *et al.* 2008; Aveyard 2014: 91–3). Unpublished literature has the disadvantage that it has not necessarily been subjected to any review, by peers or editors, which can mean that it has not been checked for certain quality standards. However, this may be less of a disadvantage than might be supposed, as you will be evaluating each paper's quality as part of the review process. The issue of whether or not the evidence has been reviewed is also not limited to whether information is published or unpublished, as published literature is itself subject to different types of review. For example, as Chapter 11 discusses, some journals require all articles to be peer reviewed prior to being accepted for publication, whilst others do not. If you decide to only include published evidence in your review, you will, therefore, also need to decide whether the published documents must be from peer reviewed sources or whether publication itself is the criteria of interest.

Whilst selecting only published literature is a common decision in literature reviews, this can significantly limit the evidence on which you base your conclusions, because not all studies publish their findings (Malicki and Marusic 2014). Siddiqi (2011) suggests that only about 50 per cent of the evidence on any given topic is published. In particular, research that reports findings that are not statistically significant, or that shows no benefit from an intervention, is less likely to be published than studies whose interventions are shown to be effective (Crombie and Davies 2009; Moreno *et al.* 2009; Hunter *et al.* 2014; Malicki and Marusic 2014). Publication bias of this type may occur because researchers choose not to report such findings, or because journals are more inclined to publish positive results (Malicki and Marusic 2014). One advantage of including unpublished literature in your review is, therefore, that it can mean that you gain a more complete set of evidence.

Nevertheless, because your study needs to be achievable, and often achievable with limited funding and within a tight time frame, a practical consideration in your decision concerning what type of literature you will include is whether or not you will be able to access the unpublished literature. Searching for and retrieving grey literature often presents more challenges than its published counterpart does. You may therefore decide that, despite the limitations of using only published literature, for practical reasons you will exclude unpublished literature from your review. You can then focus on searching systematically and rigorously for the published literature related to your question, rather than trying to include some grey literature, but without any certainty as to how effectively you will achieve this. As with all decisions about your review, the key thing is to ensure that the decisions made are clear, justified, contribute to the review being systematic, rigorous and unbiased, and that the strengths and limitations of the decisions made are acknowledged.

6.3.2 Other inclusion and exclusion criteria

The keywords that you develop for your search are likely to include the population, sample or setting that you are interested in. This is, nonetheless, worth restating in your inclusion and exclusion criteria, so that there is absolute clarity about what flexibility, if any, existed regarding this aspect of your review. In the case of the question:

> Is using a recorded handover as effective as using a face-to-face handover for nurses on acute wards?

the population would be nurses on acute wards. Your inclusion criteria would therefore state 'nurses' and the exclusion criteria 'any group of people other than nurses'. A further inclusion criterion would be acute wards, with the exclusion criteria including: community-based handovers, long stay wards, rehabilitation wards, outpatient departments.

A further consideration in the inclusion and exclusion criteria is the age of the evidence that you will consider. The dates of the literature that you are interested in can usually be entered into your search, and using this function avoids obtaining information that you know you will not use. A common recommendation is that, in order to ensure that you have the current best evidence, you should exclude literature that was published (or made available if it is unpublished) more than five (or at most ten) years ago (Cronin *et al.* 2008; Kamienski *et al.* 2013). There may, however, be times when this general recommendation does not apply. These might include situations where you want to include historical insights that are relevant to your question, or if a highly significant gold standard study was carried out at an earlier date. The decision you make about the age of the literature that you include in your review should be based on the question you want to answer, and be justifiable. In some cases this will be five to ten years, in others it may, for specific reasons that should be explained, be longer.

Depending on your study question, it may be appropriate for you to only review the evidence related to a particular region or country. In other instances, the right decision could be to evaluate the evidence from any country in the world. This decision might be based on your expectations of the applicability of information. If you are evaluating the evidence related to recorded nursing handovers, your decision could be that evidence from any country would be equally applicable. However, if you were exploring something that you thought would involve considerable variation between countries, because of geographical, cultural or health policy differences, you might decide to restrict the search to evidence from the country that you practice in. You might even decide to limit the evidence to a particular region in a country, for example to rural or urban areas. If you were, say, interested in information relevant specifically to rural Australia, your inclusion criteria might state that you would include literature related to rural areas of Australia, and exclude literature pertaining to urban areas of Australia, and all countries other than Australia.

These decisions will, again, be based in part on what should ideally be included in a review on the subject in question, but also in part on practicalities. If a vast range of research concerning a particular subject seems likely to exist, and you have limited time and funding to conduct your review, you may decide to limit your study to literature from the country where you work, even if international perspectives might also be relevant. This could be justifiable because it would enable you to rigorously and systematically find, evaluate and synthesize all the literature within your inclusion and exclusion criteria. This would be preferable to attempting to carry out a study which included more but consequently lacked system and rigour. The decision is yours to make, but the reason for it, and the implications of your choice for the review, should be clear.

The language in which the documents you will review is written is a further decision that you will need to make, and again one which you can often specify in your search. In some reviews (especially large, well-funded reviews), no language limitations are necessary, as translators can be made available. However, if you have no funding for translation, you should limit your search to information that is written in languages that you understand well enough to be able to critically evaluate the literature that you retrieve.

Developing the inclusion and exclusion criteria for your study will enable you to devise a clear statement regarding what literature you will and will not include in the documents that you review. For example, for the question: 'Is using a recorded handover as effective as using a face-to-face handover for nurses on acute wards?' the inclusion and exclusion criteria that might be developed are shown in Box 6.2:

Box 6.2

Inclusion and exclusion criteria

Is using a recorded handover as effective as using a face-to-face handover for nurses on acute wards?

Inclusion criteria: research, published literature, last five years, English language, literature from any country, literature about nurses.

Exclusion criteria: any literature that does not report original research, unpublished literature, literature older than five years, literature in languages other than English, literature related to any profession other than nursing.

Pitfall to avoid

Be realistic about what you can achieve in the time and with the resources that you have to conduct your literature review. Make sure that your inclusion and exclusion criteria are achievable, justifiable, and such that your study will remain rigorous, systematic and unbiased.

Having decided on your key terms, how you will use Boolean operators, the fields you will search in, and what your inclusion and exclusion criteria will be, you need to decide where you will look for information.

6.4 Where to search for information

The best place to look for information depends on what information you want, and links with the decisions that you made about the study's inclusion and exclusion criteria (such as whether you only intend to use published literature, or whether you will also use evidence drawn from the grey literature).

You will almost certainly want to include published literature in your review, so a part of your search strategy will be to identify relevant bibliographic databases (file structures that can be searched) of published material (Hebda and Czar 2009). Different databases deal with different subject material, so you will need to decide which databases are likely to contain information relevant to the subject that you are studying (Cronin *et al.* 2008). As the review should aim to gather all the available information related to the study question, the databases selected should be all those that cover the relevant subject areas (Cronin *et al.* 2008). There are many databases that are likely to be useful for you to consider, some of which are shown in Box 6.3.

Healthcare organizations and universities usually have subscriptions to a range of databases, which enable you to access the full text of many articles online. However, there may still be some articles that are relevant to your review whose full text is not included in your organization's subscription, and for which you will need to apply for an interlibrary loan. Although these loans are often now delivered electronically, when you plan the time schedule for your review, you should take into account the possibility of needing to wait for interlibrary loans to arrive.

In addition to individual databases, you may be able to access electronic portals that allow you to search more than one database at a time. For instance, OpenAthens (www.openathens.net) allows you to access a range of databases and electronic resources through one sign-in process. You still need to check that the databases contained within a particular portal are the ones that you want to use, but such portals are often a very convenient way to access a number of databases in one go. If you were seeking literature on recorded nursing handovers, you might have identified that some of the databases that would probably have evidence on this subject would be the British Nursing Index, CINAHL and MEDLINE. Therefore, before using a particular electronic portal you would need to check that it included those databases.

Box 6.3

Useful databases

CINAHL (The Cumulative Index to Nursing and Allied Health Literature)

EMBASE (a database of biomedical literature)

AMED (a database dedicated to allied and complementary medicine)

British Nursing Index (a database of UK-based nursing and midwifery information)

HMIC (The database of the Health Management Information Consortium)

MEDLINE (a database of biomedical literature)

PsycINFO (a database related to psychology, behavioural and social sciences)

Search engines can also be used to seek information for a literature review, but they are slightly different from databases. They search every page on every website that they have access to, looking for information related to your request (Saba and McCormick 2001). Some search engines do this for the content of a large portion of the World Wide Web. For instance, general search engines such as Google search a combination of websites, links to scholarly literature and advertisements. The results that Google returns to you are, in part, presented according to the popularity of the items that the search engine finds (Brazabon 2007; Bannigan and Spring 2015). Google Scholar focuses on scholarly literature, but still tends to present the results in terms of what the most popular results are, and what is available online, in full text format (Bannigan and Spring 2015; Waltho *et al.* 2015). In contrast, specialized search engines are selective about what part of the Web they look at, and individual websites often use a search engine that only looks at the content of their own site. Box 6.4 lists some specialized websites that can be very useful to use when you are searching for good quality health-related information.

Search engines can therefore be a useful way of finding information, but how valuable they are for searching for information for your literature review depends on what you want to find, and which search engine you use. Because search engines only collect items that they find on web pages, they will not necessarily provide you with a list of articles that is as comprehensive as that provided by a database of journal articles (Waltho *et al.* 2015). In contrast, bibliographic databases only focus on published literature, so if your inclusion criteria encompass the grey literature, search engines can be very useful. Similarly, if you know exactly what you are looking for (for example, a specific article), Google Scholar can provide very good, full text results (Waltho *et al.* 2015). Conversely, if you do not know exactly which article you are searching for, and need a system that will focus

---

Box 6.4

Examples of specialist websites

Cochrane: www.cochrane.org

ProQuest Dissertations and Theses (also known as the Index to Theses): www.theses.com

The Joanna Briggs Institute: http://joannabriggs.org

The National Institutes of Health: www.nih.gov

The National Institute for Health and Care Excellence (NICE): www.nice.org.uk

on the keywords that you are interested in, a bibliographic database will probably better suit your needs (Bannigan and Spring 2015).

The focus in discussions of searching for literature is often on the relative merits of various electronic sources. However, very few electronic searches are completely free from human or technological error. It can, therefore, also be very useful to use non-electronic sources in your quest for information. Reference chaining (cross-checking the reference lists of the articles you have retrieved using electronic sources) to check that you have not inadvertently omitted anything relevant is one method that can be used (Levy and Ellis 2006; Cronin *et al.* 2008; Aveyard 2014: 91–3; Golder *et al.* 2014). Another option is to browse the content lists of any specialist journals related to your subject area, to reduce the chance of missing useful articles.

Your decision about whether or not to move outside the use of bibliographic databases therefore really rests on what type of information you are looking for, as defined in your inclusion and exclusion criteria. Often, your search should include more than one approach. For instance, if you decided to use only published material in your review you would probably start by searching the relevant bibliographic databases. You could then use reference chaining from the documents that you found to ensure that you had not missed anything. In addition, if your inclusion criteria encompassed systematic reviews, it would be expedient to include a search of Cochrane and the Joanna Briggs Institute databases to check whether any reviews had been published there that were not highlighted using the other search options.

Once you have identified how you will carry out your search, the next step is to perform the search, retrieve the literature and record your initial results.

Pitfall to avoid

In most cases, it is expedient to avoid relying completely on one approach to searching.

6.5 The practicalities of searching and recording the results of the search

Having decided on the format for your search, and where you will search, you need to follow the instructions that you have developed, carry out the search or searches that this requires, and record the results. If you record what you find as you carry out each part of each search you will avoid having to repeat the searches later on, and will, by so doing, make the process that your study follows more systematic and rigorous.

For each search that you perform, you should record:

- where you searched;
- how you searched (for example the keywords, Boolean operators, dates and other limiters that you used);
- how many results you obtained;
- how many of these results you selected as potentially relevant for the review;
- how many documents you rejected (and why they were rejected);
- how many documents therefore remained.

As you continue your search for literature to include in the review, you also need to note how many duplicate documents your searches return (for example, you will often find the same article on two databases).

Having conducted the searches that you planned, and recorded the results, you should peruse the documents you have obtained, checking them against your inclusion and exclusion criteria, to see whether they should all become data for your review. If any of the documents do not, on closer inspection, meet the inclusion criteria, or if they fall within the exclusion criteria, they should be excluded. The number of documents excluded at this stage, and the reason for their exclusion, should be noted.

This process will give you your final list of all the articles that will be included in your review, and a clear, logical record of those that were excluded, why they were excluded, and how you have ended up with the number that you have.

If your initial search does not return as many results as you thought it would, you may need to work back through your decisions, to see if there are any sources of information, such as additional databases, that you have not included. If revising this step reveals no additional documents, you should return to your search terms and see if there are any keywords or synonyms that you have omitted. Revisiting the decisions you made about Boolean operators, especially the 'not' operator, can also be helpful, to ensure that you have not inadvertently excluded studies that might contain relevant evidence. You can also check that you have not searched in too narrow a field, for example, if you have only searched in the document title you could expand this to the title, abstract and keywords. Alternatively, if you are confident that you really have gathered all the available evidence related to your intended search, but feel that this is not enough to carry out a literature review, you may need to revisit your decisions and widen your search. For instance, you may decide to include more types of literature, more locations or a wider time frame. If you still have very little evidence, you may need to return to your review question and consider making this slightly broader.

Alternatively, if you have an excessive number of papers, beyond what you will be able to meaningfully sift through, you should consider whether your search was focused enough. This includes revisiting the decisions you made concerning your keywords and synonyms, checking whether you have made the best use of Boolean operators, and whether you have searched in the right field. If you have ensured that all of this is as good as it can be, but you still have a volume of literature that will make for an unmanageable study, you should consider how you might narrow your focus without reducing the system and rigour of your search. This could be by revisiting the inclusion and exclusion criteria, perhaps narrowing the type of literature you are interested in, the date range you are interested in, and the language or location of studies. If you still have too many results to be manageable, you may need to revise your review question to be more specific.

It is usually useful to create a table or diagram to illustrate the process of your search (Kamienski *et al.* 2013). This will provide your reader with an at-a-glance view of how you acquired the data for your review, and will help them to follow your decision trail. You can also, at this point, start to create a table with headings such as: the article title; year of publication; journal title; topic; and type of study, which can be built upon as you appraise the individual studies. This commences the process of data extraction, whereby you extract the information you need from each article, but also appraise its quality, so as to have a clear and easy-to-follow summary of your sources of information and initial findings. The sooner you begin this process, the easier it is to ensure that everything you do is recorded, and that your reader ultimately has a clear picture of how you conducted your study, what you found, and can see that the process was systematic and rigorous.

Summary

The process of searching for the literature that you will include in your review should be logical, systematic, rigorous and unbiased. In addition, the manner in which you document this should convince your reader that you have retrieved all the information that was relevant to your review question. The searching process should include: developing key concepts and from these identifying keywords and their synonyms; deciding how to use Boolean operators; creating inclusion and exclusion criteria; and deciding where you will search. Having made these decisions, your search can be performed, and the results of each stage of your search recorded. Once you have retrieved the literature that you will review, the next stage is to read it and decide on its quality.

Terminology

Boolean logic: a system that enables you to search for particular combinations of keywords or concepts in a single search.

Databases: file structures that can be searched.

Exclusion criteria: criteria that would make literature ineligible for inclusion in a review.

Grey literature: unpublished literature.

Inclusion criteria: the criteria that literature must meet in order to be included in a review.

Keywords/key concepts: the words or concepts that are crucial to your review question.

Search engine: electronic processes that enable all or parts of the World Wide Web to be searched.

Synonyms: words that mean the same as the review's keywords or concepts.

Key points:

- The process of appraising each individual piece of evidence that will be included in a literature review should be systematic and rigorous.
- Using an appropriate critical appraisal tool can assist in ensuring that each piece of evidence is evaluated consistently, and that no important issues are omitted.
- Qualitative, quantitative and mixed methods research have many similarities, but also important differences, which must be taken into account when appraising studies.
- Non-research evidence should be appraised using criteria appropriate to the type of evidence in question.

Having gathered the existing literature on a subject, the next stage in the process of conducting a study that uses literature review methodology is to appraise the quality of each piece of evidence that you have gathered. This evaluation should follow a process that is rigorous, systematic, unbiased and appropriate for the type of evidence in question.

7.1 The process of appraising the literature

Before you begin the process of carrying out a detailed evaluation of the documents that you think will be included in your review, it is useful to read through each one in order to form a general impression of it. Even with a very focused search it is quite common for one or two of the documents that you obtain either to not concern exactly the subject that their title, keywords and abstract suggest, or to not meet your inclusion and exclusion criteria. It is therefore worth reading all the papers that you have retrieved and making any further exclusions that you consider necessary before beginning the formal appraisal of them. Any exclusions that you make at this point, and the reason for your decision, should be noted, so that your reader can understand the process that you followed and see that it was systematic, rigorous and unbiased.

Pitfall to avoid

Do not exclude any papers without making a note of what you excluded, and why you excluded it.

Carrying out an initial perusal of all the documents that you have gathered allows you to determine the range of evidence that you have, and to gain some initial impressions of its quality. As you do this, it is useful to make some notes (in a table or whatever format you find works best for you) about each paper, including information such as (Cronin *et al.* 2008):

- author name;
- year of publication;
- title of the paper;
- aim of the paper;
- type of evidence;
- key findings;
- conclusions.

This information will be useful to have to hand later on, as you develop your in-depth analysis of each paper, and subsequently collate the findings from across sources (as described in Chapter 8). It also enables you to plan the practicalities of how you will carry out the appraisal of all the literature that you have gathered, for instance whether you will appraise all the qualitative research papers, then all the quantitative research papers, etc. This initial reading and organizing of the papers must then be followed by an in-depth critical appraisal of each document (Cronin *et al.* 2008).

The process of critical appraisal involves carefully and systematically examining each piece of literature that you have obtained in order to judge its quality (Burls 2009). This means identifying the paper's strengths and limitations, and deciding how important each of these factors is in determining the overall quality of the evidence presented. The criteria that you use to make these judgements will depend on the nature of the literature, but your decisions should be reached by rigorous, systematic, consistent and unbiased means

(Cronin *et al.* 2008; Hemingway and Brereton 2009; Murphy *et al.* 2009).

Where the papers that you are evaluating report on research, there are established quality indicators that can be used to guide your appraisal of them (Hemingway and Brereton 2009). Some general principles that can be used to appraise the rigour and system of any type of research are shown in Box 7.1. However, the precise criteria that you should use to appraise the methodological quality of a study will depend on the type of research in question.

Box 7.1

Principles that can be used to evaluate research

- Does the study have a clear purpose or aim?
- Is there evidence of a sound rationale for the study being undertaken, including an objective review of the relevant literature? (Achieving this suggests that the researcher was unbiased, up to date, and understood the subject sufficiently well to study it.)
- Do the background and rationale for the study relate to the study purpose/question/aims? (This is one indicator of whether or not the study appears to follow a systematic process.)
- Is the study paradigm or methodology appropriate for the subject being investigated? (For the study to be rigorous and systematic, the paradigm or methodology used should be consistent with the study purpose/question/aims, and be reflected in all the decisions made about the methods of data collection and analysis.)
- Were appropriate data collection methods used? (The methods used should be consistent with the methodology, and suitable for gathering information that would address the study purpose/question/aims.)
- Would the sampling processes used have ensured that the right type and quality of data were gathered? Were they consistent with the study aims, methodology and methods?
- Were data analysed using processes that matched the study purpose/question/aims, methodology, and type of data gathered?
- Were the results or findings presented clearly and logically? Were they related to the study purpose/question/aims? Were they derived from processes described in the study methods? (For the study to be systematic and rigorous, there should be no unexplained gaps in the findings, or findings that do not seem to proceed from any process described in the methodology and methods.)

- Was there a discussion of the findings? (A discussion of the findings shows how these relate to the existing evidence in the field, and contextualizes them within the study as a whole.)
- Do the conclusions and recommendations address the study question and aims, fit the research paradigm or methodology, and arise directly from the study findings? (In order for a study to be logical, systematic and rigorous, and for its claims to be justifiable, a study's conclusions and recommendations should be derived from the findings.)
- Did the study conform to the ethical principles of doing good (beneficence), doing no harm (non-maleficence), respecting autonomy and seeking justice (Beauchamp and Childress 2013)?

There are a number of critical appraisal tools that provide guidance on how to evaluate various types of research. These can be very useful in assisting you to make your appraisal systematic and structured, and to ensure that you consider all the key quality issues relevant to the type of research that you are evaluating (Aveyard 2014: 110). In addition, using the same appraisal tool for all the studies of a particular design or methodology contributes to the judgements you make being consistent and unbiased across papers. One such set of tools are the Critical Appraisal Skills Programme (CASP project) tools, which are available at: www.casp-uk.net/#!checklists/cb36.

Whilst such tools or checklists are very useful, you need to ensure that any that you employ are appropriate for the design and methodology of the studies that you use them for. If not, regardless of the intrinsic value of the tool, you will not be using a valid measure to assess the quality of the paper in question. If, for example, you evaluated a qualitative study using the CASP tool for randomized controlled trials, you would end up judging the study to be of very poor quality. However, this would not be a reasonable judgement, as the quality criteria for qualitative research and randomized controlled trials are very different. Thus, despite the CASP tool for randomized controlled trials being a high-quality evaluation tool, it would not be a valid choice for this task. An appropriate choice would be the CASP tool for qualitative studies. As you appraise each paper that is included in your review key issues to consider are therefore the type of evidence that you are evaluating, and to what extent the quality criteria for this kind of evidence have been met.

> **Pitfall to avoid**
>
> Ensure that any evaluation tool you use is itself of good quality, and that you are using it to appraise the type of evidence that it was designed to assess.

7.2 Appraising quantitative research

The paradigm (or belief that underpins) quantitative research (also sometimes referred to as positivist research) is that truth is objective, not dependent on context or interpretation, and that one can determine (using statistics), whether or not something will usually work for a given population (Ross 2012: 35–6; Claydon 2015). A key aim of quantitative research is therefore to produce generalizable results: findings that can be applied equally to most people within a certain population or group. Consequently, a major issue in determining the quality of quantitative research is how far a study's findings can be generalized (Ross 2012: 35–6). For instance, a quantitative study aimed at ascertaining whether taking 20 minutes of exercise daily assists people aged over 65 to lose weight would ideally determine whether or not this would be the case for the vast majority of people aged over 65 in a given population.

The two main quality indicators that influence whether or not a quantitative study achieves generalizability are reliability and validity (Heale and Twycross 2015). Evaluating a quantitative study therefore usually focuses on determining how far these criteria have been met.

7.2.1 Reliability and validity

The reliability of a study concerns whether the way in which it was designed and conducted means that it will have accurately and consistently addressed the research aim and measured what it was intended to measure (Wilson and Gochyyev 2013; Heale and Twycross 2015). If a study is deemed to be reliable it means that there is confidence that the results that it reports are due to what was being investigated, rather than because of an error in some part of the research process. There can therefore be confidence that if it were repeated it would produce similar results, assuming that nothing else had changed (Heale and Twycross 2015). A study might report that undertaking 20 minutes of exercise daily for a 6-month period was associated with people aged over 65 consistently losing weight. If the study was reliable, the same result would be found if it was repeated using identical methods and sampling strategies.

Validity refers to whether what was intended to be measured in a study is what was actually measured (Heale and Twycross 2015; Wilson and Gochyyev 2013). Specific types of validity have been described, four of which are shown in Box 7.2. It is also common to see validity described as being divided into internal and external validity. Internal validity concerns whether or not there could have been reasons other than the issue being investigated for the apparent outcomes of a study (Roberts and Priest 2006). For instance, for a study concerning the effects of people aged over 65 undertaking exercise to achieve internal validity it would be necessary to ensure that other factors (such as diet, specific health issues, other changes in lifestyle) would not have influenced the study outcomes. Internal validity is also reliant on a study being designed and conducted in a manner that ensures that what it claims to investigate is what was actually studied (Roberts and Priest 2006; Maltby *et al.* 2010). External validity relates to how far the study's findings can be applied externally (its generalizability) (Roberts and Priest 2006; Maltby *et al.* 2010).

Box 7.2

Types of validity

Face validity: the extent to which the tools used in a study measure what they claim to measure.

Content validity: how accurately the tools used in a study reflect the existing literature on the subject (this can only be achieved if such literature exists).

Criterion validity: how the measures used in the study compare or relate to established measures.

Construct validity: whether the instrument(s) used in the study really measure what they claim to measure.

(Jack *et al.* 2010; Ross 2012; Jones and Rattray 2015)

Each decision made regarding the design and conduct of a study will affect how valid and reliable it is, and thus its quality. Some key issues to consider when evaluating a quantitative study, alongside the general quality indicators for research highlighted in Box 7.1, include the following:

7.2.2 The focus of the study

Quantitative studies usually have a research question or hypothesis (Ross 2012). Box 7.3 outlines the attributes and uses of a hypothesis, but if the intention of a study is to conduct an experiment designed to establish cause and effect, a hypothesis should usually be used to state the focus of the research. A study investigating whether undertaking twenty minutes of exercise each day enables people aged over 65 to lose weight might state the hypothesis: '20 minutes a day of exercise assists people aged over 65 to lose weight'. The aim of the study would then be to demonstrate whether or not this hypothesis was upheld.

Box 7.3

Hypotheses

A hypothesis: a statement about the association between variables. The hypothesis is either upheld or not depending on the results of the study.

The Alternate Hypothesis (usually referred to as 'the hypothesis'): a statement of positive association or effect between variables, e.g.: twenty minutes of exercise each day is associated with weight loss.

The Null Hypothesis: a statement of no effect or no association between variables (Ren 2009), e.g.: there is no association between undertaking twenty minutes of exercise each day and weight loss.

How the hypotheses work: statistically, a study's hypothesis is upheld by refuting the null hypothesis (Ren 2009). The null hypothesis is therefore tested and upheld or not, and, by association, the hypothesis (which is its direct opposite) is either upheld or not.

However, not all quantitative research is suitable for hypothesis testing. Studies that do not aim to show cause and effect or to demonstrate something beyond reasonable doubt usually instead refer to the purpose of the study, the research problem, or question. If you are evaluating a quantitative study, the key issue to determine is whether there is a clear statement regarding the intention of the research, and whether the way that this is presented is congruent with the nature of the study.

Pitfall to avoid

Do not assume that a quantitative study always needs a hypothesis, or will be improved by having one. What matters is whether the study has a clear focus that is stated in a manner appropriate to the nature of the research.

7.2.3 The study design

The quantitative research paradigm encompasses a number of different study designs that fall within two broad categories: experimental and non-experimental (also referred to as observational or descriptive) studies (Tolmie *et al.* 2011; Ross 2012). Whilst some study designs are, in principle, better at producing generalizable results than others, when you evaluate a study what is important is to determine whether the chosen design is consistent with the study aim, question or hypothesis. Having a research design that matches the study question, aim or hypothesis provides an early indication that the study has an element of consistency, system and rigour. In contrast, using a design that is, in principle, very good at achieving generalizable results but which is not appropriate for addressing a particular study question or aim will not produce a good quality study.

The intention of experimental studies is to identify cause and effect relationships (Tolmie *et al.* 2011). In order to achieve this, they should be designed so as to create as much certainty as possible that any effect seen is due to what is being tested, not something else (Allen *et al.* 2009; Tolmie *et al.* 2011). The study design should, therefore, allow what is being tested to be effectively isolated from other factors. An experiment designed to test whether exercising for twenty minutes a day enabled people aged over sixty-five to lose weight would need to isolate exercise from all other factors, so as to be sure that only the effect of exercise was being evaluated.

Studies that use an experimental design almost always have a hypothesis, because the researcher is trying to show whether there is an association between what is being tested and a particular outcome. Here are some particular design considerations that should be included in an evaluation of an experimental study:

- Was the experiment designed in a way that would ensure that it effectively tested or compared what it said it did (to achieve reliability and validity)?
- Was there a control group (a group that either has no intervention at all, or the intervention that they would have had if the experiment was not happening)? This provides something against which the effect of the intervention can be compared (Parahoo 2014).
- Were the control and intervention groups as exact a match as possible (in terms of key factors such as age, sex and diagnosis (Parahoo 2014)? This assists in achieving internal validity by ensuring that the only difference between the two groups is what is being studied.

- If an intervention and control group were used, were participants randomly allocated to one group or another (Parahoo 2014)? This contributes to the study's validity by ensuring that there was no reason other than chance for any participant to be allocated to either group. Therefore any differences in the findings between the groups would be likely be due to the intervention, not other factors. A randomized controlled trial comparing weight loss in people aged over 65 who exercised daily and those who did not would allocate individuals to the group who exercised and the group who did not exercise using random sampling. This would mean that there was an equal chance of every person in the study population being allocated to either group.
- Was blinding (see Box 7.4) used where appropriate? This can add to the study's reliability and validity by removing the possibility of the results being affected by people knowing who was in each study group. However, blinding is not always possible or appropriate. For example, in an experiment to assess whether undertaking twenty minutes of exercise a day resulted in weight loss, it would not be possible to blind participants to whether or not they undertook exercise.

Whilst experimental studies (such as a randomized controlled trial) are often seen as the pinnacle of quantitative research, there are many instances where quantitative enquiry is appropriate, but where an

---

Box 7.4

Blinding

Blinding: the study group that individuals have been allocated to is not known (for example, whether they have been allocated to receive an experimental drug or a placebo). This prevents the outcome of the experiment being influenced by individuals knowing which group particular participants are in (Nelson *et al.* 2015).

Single blinding: the research participant does not know which group they are in, but the researcher knows which person has which intervention. With single blinding, the researcher knowing which group participants are in could result in them inadvertently treating them differently, or interpreting their results in a particular way.

Double blinding: neither the researcher nor the person involved in the experiment knows which study group they are in (Nelson *et al.* 2015).

experiment is not possible. In such situations non-experimental study designs can be used, examples of which are shown in Box 7.5. These, like all research, should be evaluated using criteria appropriate for the study design in question.

Box 7.5

Observational or descriptive studies

Case control studies:

Individuals who are receiving the intervention of interest or have developed the disease or condition of interest are identified. These people are the cases.

Controls are found who are as close a match as possible for these cases in terms of key characteristics (such as diagnosis, age and sex) but who did not receive the intervention or develop the disease or condition. The outcomes of interest for the cases and controls are compared (Hoe and Hoare 2012).

Longitudinal/cohort studies:

Individuals who have something of interest to the researcher are followed over time with data collected at two or more points (Hoe and Hoare 2012).

Cross-sectional studies:

Studies that are carried out at one point in time and provide a snapshot of whatever is of interest (Jack *et al.* 2010; Hasson *et al.* 2015).

Pitfall to avoid

Do not assume that an experimental study is always the best design for quantitative research. What is important is whether the study design would have enabled the focus of the research to be addressed, and the aim(s) to be achieved.

7.2.4 Sampling

Probability (or random) sampling is often considered the best method of sampling in quantitative research, as it has the greatest likelihood of achieving generalizability (Tolmie *et al.* 2011). The principle of probability sampling is that once the population that is being studied has been determined, everyone in that population has an equal chance of being selected for the study (Tolmie *et al.* 2011). Because each person could equally have been a research subject, the results of the study should, theoretically, be generalizable to anyone in that population. Using probability sampling therefore contributes to a study achieving external validity (Maltby *et al.* 2010). It also contributes to achieving internal validity, by reducing the risk of factors such as the individual characteristics of participants having an effect on the study outcomes (as any member of the population had an equal chance of being selected).

Non-probability sampling strategies (see Box 7.6) are not generally considered to be as good as probability sampling for quantitative research, because all members of the population do not have an equal chance of being included (Tolmie *et al.* 2011). As a result they do not produce results that can be as confidently generalized. However, probability sampling cannot always be achieved and in some cases is not appropriate for the study question, aim or design. When you are evaluating a quantitative study the key issues to consider related to how the sample were selected are:

- Was probability sampling used?
- If not, what approach was used?
- What would the effects of this have been on the quality of the study?
- Were the strengths and limitations of the sampling strategy used reflected in the claims made about the study findings?

The size of the sample is also an important consideration in any research. As the intention of quantitative research is generalize to an entire population the ideal is for the sample to be large enough to make this possible. Often, a sample size formula (or power calculation) is used to determine the sample size that is required to achieve

---

Box 7.6

Types of non-probability sampling

Purposive sampling: the research participants are selected on purpose because they are considered likely to provide the most comprehensive data concerning the matter under investigation (Hunt and Lathlean 2015).

Snowball sampling: the initial research participants refer the researcher to other potential participants (Hunt and Lathlean 2015).

Convenience sampling: the research participants are the people who are available or accessible at the time in question (Hunt and Lathlean 2015).

generalizability (Jack *et al.* 2010; Maltby *et al.* 2010). When you are evaluating a quantitative paper, two important questions related to the sample size are:

• How large was the sample size?
• How did the researchers know whether or not this was a large enough number to produce generalizable results?

Although a sample size formula can be used to determine how many participants are needed for a study to achieve generalizability, in some cases recruiting people to a study does not guarantee that they will participate. In such instances (for example, where a questionnaire is distributed with no guarantee of return), the number of those who participated, as well as those who were in the original sample, needs to be noted. A low uptake, or response rate, reduces the chance of the sample being representative of the population studied and therefore the generalizability of the study's findings (Ross 2012). There is not absolute agreement on what an adequate response rate is: Burns and Grove (2005) and Polit and Beck (2006) suggest 50 per cent as the level below which the quality of the research findings might be questionable, whilst 60 per cent has also been suggested as the lower end of acceptable response rates (Finchman 2008).

The main issues to consider when evaluating the sampling strategy for a quantitative study are therefore:

• Was the right, or best possible, method of sampling used for the study in question?
• What effect would the sampling strategy have had on the reliability and validity of the study?
• Was the sample large enough to be expected to produce generalizable results?
• (Where relevant) was the response rate adequate?

7.2.5 Study methods

There are numerous methods of gathering quantitative data, none of which is inherently superior to another. In terms of study quality, what matters is whether the methods used would have accurately and consistently gathered the right type of data to address the study hypothesis, question or aims.

How the reliability and validity of the methods used in a study should be assessed depends on what these are. For example, a study designed to assess whether or not twenty minutes of exercise per day influenced weight loss would have to use a method of measuring the duration of people's exercise that would consistently and accurately record this information. People's weight would also need to be assessed using a method that was reliable and valid.

Questionnaires are a very commonly used method in quantitative research. For a study that uses a questionnaire as a method of collecting data to be reliable and valid there are certain aspects of the design and conduct of the questionnaire that should be considered, some of which are shown in Box 7.7.

7.2.6 Data analysis

As the intention of quantitative research is to numerically evaluate facts, data are analysed using statistical tests. When you evaluate the way in which data in a quantitative study were analysed you should therefore determine whether the right statistical tests have to be applied to the data in question. If the wrong tests have been used, the apparent findings will not be reliable or valid, because what the study intended to measure will not have been represented accurately.

Box 7.7

Evaluating the reliability and validity of questionnaires

Reliability:
- Do the questions address the research question and aim(s)?
- Would everyone interpret the questions in the same way?
- Has the questionnaire been tested or used previously?
- Does the questionnaire use an accepted or standardized test or scale?
- Were subject experts involved in the development of the questionnaire?
- Was the questionnaire piloted?

Validity:
- Does the questionnaire measure what it is supposed to measure, or obtain the right type of information?
- Was a comprehensive literature review used to guide the content of the questionnaire?
- Was the questionnaire piloted?
- Was the questionnaire compared to validated measures of the same concept or phenomenon (this can only be done when other such measures exist)?

(Maltby *et al*. 2010)

In order to determine whether or not the right statistical test has been used, it is first necessary to ascertain what type of data the study generated. This involves deciding whether the data were parametric or non-parametric (see Box 7.8). Parametric data can be analysed using either parametric or non-parametric tests, although they are usually evaluated using parametric tests as these are more powerful (better at detecting small differences between groups). Non-parametric data should only be analysed using non-parametric tests. Although non-parametric tests are generally less powerful than parametric tests, in terms of study quality what matters is that the right test was used for the type of data in question. Using parametric tests to analyse non-parametric data would therefore significantly detract from study quality, despite these tests being, in principle, more powerful.

Box 7.8

The characteristics of parametric and non-parametric data

Parametric data:

- The observations/data that are collected are independent of all other observations or data.
- The data follow a normal distribution curve (if the data were displayed as a graph they would form a bell-shaped curve).
- Interval or ratio data are used. Interval and ratio data are measurements that form part of a scale in which each position is the same distance from the next. For example, the difference between 1 cm and 2 cm is the same as between 2 cm and 3 cm. In interval data an absolute zero score does not exist, whereas in ratio data it does. As such, temperature measurements are interval data, as temperatures may be below zero, whereas weight is usually regarded as ratio data as a person cannot weigh less than 0 kg (Maltby *et al.* 2010; Ross 2012).

Non-parametric data:

- The data do not follow a normal distribution curve.
- Nominal or ordinal data are used. Nominal data use a system that has no numerical meaning, for example a person's sex. Ordinal data use numbers and can be placed in order to show their relative position, but there is not the same measurable difference between each point on the scale. Satisfaction scales and pay grades are examples of ordinal data.
- The sample size is small (Maltby *et al.* 2010; Greenhalgh 2010; Ross 2012).

Having decided whether particular data should have been analysed using parametric or non-parametric tests, which specific tests were used and whether these were appropriate then needs to be checked. There are two broad divisions of statistical tests: descriptive statistics and inferential statistics (Maltby *et al.* 2010: 207; Ross 2012). Descriptive statistics (percentage, median, mean and mode scores) are used to describe the data that have been gathered and summarize this. The median (the value at the precise middle when all the values are arranged in numerical order), mean (average) and mode (value that occurs most frequently) can also be used to calculate the central tendency (central value) of the data (Ross 2012). The descriptive statistical tests that can be applied to particular types of data are shown in Box 7.9.

The studies that you evaluate may also show the spread (or dispersion) that exists around the central tendency in order to show the range that the data covers, as well as the midpoint score (Tolmie *et al.* 2011). This information can be useful as it provides an indication of whether the results were clustered around the midpoint, or whether there was considerable variation from this value. For example, a study might show that the mean weight loss for people aged over sixty-five who undertook twenty minutes of exercise each day was 6 kg over six months. However, the measure of dispersion would show whether the weight lost ranged from a gain of 10 kg to a loss of 10 kg, or was mostly clustered around the 6 kg loss value. Measures of dispersion that are commonly used are:

- Standard deviation: shows how much variation there is from the mean, and can therefore only be used for parametric data as non-parametric data do not have a mean value (Tolmie *et al.* 2011; Ross 2012).

Box 7.9

Descriptive statistical tests

Parametric data: percentage, mean, median or mode can be used (Tolmie *et al.* 2011; Ross 2012).

Non-parametric data:
- Ordinal data: percentage, median or mode can be used (Tolmie *et al.* 2011). (A mean value cannot be calculated because there is not the same measurable difference between each point on a scale that uses ordinal data.)
- Nominal data: percentage or mode can be used (Tolmie *et al.* 2011) (Nominal data does not have a numerical value therefore a mean or median score cannot be calculated.)

- Interquartile range: is used for ordinal data (Tolmie *et al.* 2011).

It is not usually appropriate to calculate measures of dispersion for nominal data as they do not have a numerical value (Tolmie *et al.* 2011). When you evaluate a study it is therefore useful to check whether any measures of dispersion were used and, if so, whether the appropriate measure was employed for the type of data in question.

These descriptive statistics provide a general idea of the findings from the sample that was studied, but they do not indicate how generalizable those findings are. To show this, inferential statistics are required. The intention of the study and whether the data gathered were parametric or non-parametric again dictates which inferential tests should be used. Some of the most commonly used tests in inferential statistics and the type of data that they should be used with are shown in Box 7.10.

Not all studies will, or should, use inferential statistical tests. For example, in a small study, from which no generalizations are intended, using only descriptive statistics is likely to be wholly appropriate. This is not a flaw in the quality of the study itself, as it achieves what it sets out to. It may, nonetheless, mean that as you form your decisions about the overall quality of the evidence that exists on your chosen subject, as described in Chapter 8, you afford it less value than findings from larger, more significant studies.

When you evaluate a quantitative study, you should check whether the statistical tests used were consistent with:

- the study aim (for example, whether the tests used were suitable for making the comparisons that the study aimed to make);
- the sample;
- the methods used;
- the type of data gathered.

7.2.7 Results

The results from quantitative research should be presented in a way that enables you to see how each set of data and the analysis of this data addressed the study question, hypothesis or aim. For instance, if a study aimed to identify whether taking twenty minutes of exercise each day enabled people aged over sixty-five to lose weight, the results should be presented in a way that focuses on whether or not this was the case.

The findings from quantitative research should usually indicate how generalizable the findings are. In some cases there will be no

Box 7.10

Commonly used inferential statistical tests

Parametric tests:

T-test: compares the mean scores from two groups.

One-sample *t*-tests compare the mean of a single group against an expected mean.

Two-sample *t*-tests compare the means of two actual groups (Nayak and Hazra 2011).

Analysis of variance (ANOVA): compares the means of more than two groups (Nayak and Hazra 2011; Martin and Bridgmon 2012).

Non-parametric tests:

Chi-square: assesses whether an outcome is likely to be due to chance, or other factors (Nayak and Hazra 2011).

Wilcoxon's test and the Mann-Whitney U test: compare the differences between two groups using median values (Nayak and Hazra 2011; Martin and Bridgmon 2012).

Kruskal-Wallis: tests for differences between the median scores of more than two groups (Nayak and Hazra 2011; Martin and Bridgmon 2012).

Correlation and regression analysis:

Correlation analysis shows the direction and strength of any relationship between two variables using values from −1.00 (a perfect negative correlation) to 1.00 (a perfect positive correlation) (Hill and Lewicki 2007; Nayak and Hazra 2011).

If correlation analysis shows a relationship between variables regression analysis can be used to make a prediction for one variable based on the value of another.

Pearson's r is a commonly used parametric correlation and regression test. Spearman's correlation is a non-parametric correlation test (Nayak and Hazra 2011).

Tailed tests:

Tailed tests specifically analyse the data that would be found at the ends of the curves on a graph (Greenhalgh 2010; Nayak and Hazra 2011). A one-tailed test analyses the information at one extreme of the graph. A two-tailed test analyses the information at both extremes.

claim to generalizability, for example where the study design has been such that only descriptive statistics were appropriate.

Inferential statistics, on the other hand, allow the expected generalizability of the study findings to be determined. However, the tests described in the previous section do not, of themselves, indicate how generalizable a result is to the population as a whole. Two ways of calculating the generalizability of the results of a statistical test are to determine the p value or the confidence interval (CI) (Ross 2012).

For the findings from a study to be considered statistically significant (or generalizable) the calculated p value should be less than 0.05 (Thomas 2005; Windish and Diener-West 2006; Ross 2012). A p value of 0.05 indicates that, statistically, there is 95 per cent certainty that the results can be generalized to the population from which the sample was drawn. The lower the p value, the more statistically significant (and the more generalizable), the findings are. A p value of 0.01 indicates 99 per cent certainty that the findings can be generalized to the population from which the sample was drawn. 95 per cent certainty is generally considered high enough for researchers to be confident about generalizing from samples to populations (Ross 2012).

A study's confidence interval (CI) also indicates how generalizable the study's findings are. It tells you how precise the result is by showing the range within which you can be confident that the result from a population from which the sample was drawn rather than just the sample tested will lie (Ross 2012). The end points of the confidence interval are referred to as confidence limits. The confidence interval is qualified by a level of confidence, usually expressed as a percentage, about the level of confidence that exists that this interval will apply to the population from which the sample was drawn. As with the p value, 95 per cent is generally considered a high enough level of confidence to make generalization appropriate (Ross 2012). A paper that reported twenty minutes a day of exercise as being associated with weight loss in people over the age of sixty-five might have a confidence interval of 15–25 minutes. If the level of confidence was stated as being 95 per cent, it would mean that there was 95 per cent confidence that all people aged over sixty-five in the general population would lose weight if they took between fifteen and twenty-five minutes exercise a day, provided nothing else changed. This would be described as the 95 per cent confidence interval being 15–25 minutes.

When you are evaluating a study, as well as checking which particular statistical tests were undertaken, you should therefore also check whether the p value and/or confidence interval were stated. If they were, you should clarify whether these indicated that the findings were generalizable (or achieved external validity), and whether any claim to generalizability made by the researchers matched this.

> **Pitfall to avoid**
>
> Avoid thinking that whether a study showed a positive outcome or achieved generalizable results is the key issue in terms of research quality. The key issue is whether the results were faithfully reported, and appropriate inferences made from these.

When you evaluate a study's results, as well as considering the results that have been presented, you should check whether there are any missing results and whether there is evidence that the researchers thought about possible alternative explanations for the results. These are sometimes described as confounding variables (things that could be the real reason for the study outcomes rather than the given reason). If you can identify possible confounding variables that were not identified and accounted for in the study, you may decide that the study's reliability and validity is limited, as issues other than those the study was investigating might have influenced the results.

Overall, then, when you evaluate a study's results, you should identify whether they address the focus of the study, and rigorously and systematically provide information on what the study set out to investigate. In addition, you should consider whether the way in which the results have been determined is reliable and valid, and whether any claims to generalizability are commensurate with the study design and findings.

7.2.8 Conclusions and recommendations

The conclusions and recommendations from a study should address the research question, hypothesis or aim (Martin and Bridgmon 2012). They should also fit the rest of the study, and should be clearly derived from, and reflect the strength of, the results (Lunenburg and Irby 2008; White 2011). For example, if the results are statistically insignificant, or if there are possible confounding variables, the conclusions and recommendations should be suitably cautious. Similarly, if only descriptive statistics have been used, generalizations should not be made.

Whilst objectivity and generalizability are the hallmarks of high-quality quantitative research, different principles underpin qualitative research, and thus the criteria for evaluating this type of research are not the same.

7.3 Appraising qualitative research

Qualitative research (sometimes referred to as research that falls within the interpretivist or naturalistic paradigm) is underpinned by very different principles from quantitative research. Its aim is to achieve in-depth understanding of issues that are likely to be subjective and individual (Pereira 2012). Because of this, the generalizability that is seen as highly desirable in quantitative enquiry is not the intention of qualitative research. It should, therefore, not be evaluated using the same criteria as quantitative research.

> **Pitfall to avoid**
>
> Do not evaluate a qualitative study using quantitative criteria.

There is not the same level of agreement about the criteria that should be used to judge the quality of qualitative research as there is for quantitative research (Jootun and McGhee 2009; De la Cuesta Benjumea 2015). However, a commonly used set of criteria are those of trustworthiness, as described by Lincoln and Guba (1985). The trustworthiness of a study in this context essentially concerns how much trust or confidence you should have that the reported findings are a true reflection of the data that were gathered in the study. Lincoln and Guba (1985) suggest that a study is likely to be trustworthy when the criteria of credibility, dependability, transferability and confirmability are met.

7.3.1 Trustworthiness

Credibility

Credibility concerns whether or not the processes of gathering and analysing data meant that the intended focus of the research was addressed (Lincoln and Guba 1985). Assessing this in a study entails evaluating whether:

- the right methods were used to gather data (Moon *et al.* 2013);
- data were gathered in adequate depth (Houghton *et al.* 2013; Moon *et al.* 2013);
- the researcher achieved prolonged engagement in the research process (to enable them to gain an in-depth understanding of the matter being investigated) (Houghton *et al.* 2013);

- data triangulation (using more than one method of gathering data to create as complete as possible a picture of the subject under investigation) was used if appropriate (Houghton *et al.* 2013);
- detailed notes were kept (Houghton *et al.* 2013);
- data were analysed using appropriate processes (Moon *et al.* 2013);
- unexpected, differing or contrasting views were presented and explored in the findings (Moon *et al.* 2013; Houghton *et al.* 2013).

The credibility of the study also rests on whether the presented findings are a faithful representation of the participants' views. Evidence of this being achieved includes:

- the researcher interpreting how their own experiences, input or presence affected the research (Pilnick and Swift 2010; Zitomer and Goodwin 2014);
- the researcher consulting with participants to check that their views have been faithfully represented (known as respondent validation or member checking) (Moon *et al.* 2013; Houghton *et al.* 2013).

Dependability (also sometimes referred to as auditability)

A study's dependability concerns whether sufficient evidence is provided about how it was conducted and how the conclusions made were reached (Moon *et al.* 2013). This can be evidenced by the researcher providing a clear and reasoned description of the study methods and processes, including how key decisions were made, for example how the codes and categories used to analyse the data were developed (Houghton *et al.* 2013).

Transferability

Qualitative research does not seek to achieve generalizability, but it is still important for a reader to know whether or not it is applicable to other situations. The concept of transferability addresses this issue, and concerns the extent to which findings can be transferred to other situations or groups. It requires the research report to give an in-depth and detailed description of the setting and context of the study, and the characteristics of participants, so that the reader can see how similar these were to the setting to which the transfer of findings is proposed (Houghton *et al.* 2013; Moon *et al.* 2013).

Confirmability

Confirmability relates to whether or not a study's apparent findings were indeed derived from the data. As such, it has links with all the other elements of trustworthiness (Lincoln and Guba 1985). Achieving confirmability is further aided by the researcher keeping a reflective journal recording their experiences, decisions, and any other potential influences on the study and its findings (Lincoln and Guba 1985).

These criteria are not universally accepted as the best way to evaluate qualitative research (Jootun and McGhee 2009; De la Cuesta Benjumea 2015). They do, however, include principles that form useful guidance as to what you should consider when you are appraising the quality of each aspect of a qualitative study.

7.3.2 The study aim

Qualitative research does not typically conduct experiments, aim to show anything beyond reasonable doubt, or to generalize findings to an entire population, therefore there is usually no study hypothesis (Ryan *et al.* 2007). However, the purpose or aim of the study should be clear, and should be appropriate for an investigation that uses qualitative methodology (Anderson 2010; Cleary *et al.* 2014). A qualitative study might, for example, aim to explore the experiences of people over sixty-five years of age who have taken up regular exercise. This aim seems suitable to address using qualitative methodology as the intention is to explore, in-depth, individual experiences, rather than to quantify something (such as the amount of weight loss achieved by undertaking exercise).

A qualitative study may be designed to answer a question, address an issue or explore a particular phenomenon. Whichever of these the study intends to achieve, the purpose of the research should be clearly stated. If it is not, it will be difficult for the research to achieve credibility because judging whether the methodology and methods used address the study's intended focus will be problematic.

7.3.3 Qualitative methodologies

Within the qualitative paradigm, there are a range of specific methodologies that can be used, the most commonly described being phenomenology, ethnography, grounded theory, and narrative research (Moon *et al.* 2013). The main principles of these methodologies are shown in Box 7.11. Some qualitative studies do not conform to any one methodological stance, whilst others combine ideas from

Box 7.11

Commonly used qualitative methodologies

Phenomenology: aims to describe people's lived experiences of what is being studied and the meaning that these experiences have for them (Willig 2008; Balls 2009; Morse 2012).

Ethnography: provides in-depth descriptions of everyday life for individuals, groups, or cultures and aims to explain how these create meaning for those involved (Morse 2012). Long-term engagement and participant observation are the mainstay of ethnography; additional data sources, such as interviews and document analysis, are often also used (Ryan *et al.* 2007).

Grounded theory: aims to develop theory about something, with the theory that is developed grounded in the data generated from the research (Holloway and Galvin 2015).

Narrative research: focuses on gathering narratives from participants that are then interpreted and analysed by the researcher and presented in a way which shows context, sequence and interpretations so that each event can be seen in relation to a whole experience (Freshwater and Holloway 2015).

more than one philosophical approach. However, a commonality between all qualitative methodologies is that they aim to gather non-numerical data, and to achieve sufficient depth of enquiry for all the intricacies of what is being explored to be understood.

When you evaluate the methodology of a qualitative study, the questions you should ask are whether this was appropriate for addressing the aim or purpose of the study, and if it would have enabled the researcher to gather in-depth data. A study might state that it used interpretive phenomenology to explore the experiences of people aged over sixty-five who began to engage in regular exercise. This would seem a suitable methodology as it would enable an in-depth exploration of people's experiences of the phenomenon of taking up exercise to be achieved.

7.3.4 Methods

Some of the most commonly used data collection methods in qualitative research are shown in Box 7.12. For a study to achieve credibility, the methods used should be consistent with the purpose of the study and its methodology, and enable in-depth data to be gathered

Box 7.12

Commonly used methods in qualitative research

Interviews:

Usually either semi-structured or unstructured (Tod 2015).

Semi-structured interviews: have a structure, and key questions or an interview schedule, but these can be adapted or developed during the interview (Tod 2015).

Unstructured interviews: are used to elicit information around a set of issues or themes. An interview guide is usually used, but there is no particular sequence or format for the questions (Tod 2015).

Interviews may be conducted: face-to-face, online or by telephone, with individuals or groups, as one-off interactions or as a series of interviews.

Observation:

Involves the researcher gaining an understanding of the people they are studying and their world by using all of their senses to witness events, note information, and then interpret this (Booth 2015).

Participant observation: the observer seeks to experience the situation which they are studying from the perspective of an insider, whilst also standing back a little to try to understand, analyse and explain it (Booth 2015).

Non-participant observation: the researcher is present but does not participate in the situation being studied (Booth 2015).

Questionnaires:

Qualitative questionnaires use open-ended questions, and their wording encourages participants to give in-depth responses.

Document analysis:

Documents may be useful as a main data source, or in building up a fuller picture of a situation that is being primarily studied by other means.

(Astin 2009; Moon *et al.* 2013; Cleary *et al.* 2014). If, for instance, a study claimed to use ethnography, but used one-off, in-depth interviews to collect data, whether this would produce ethnographic data would be questionable. In contrast, for a study that claimed to use phenomenology, using one-off, in-depth interviews would often be entirely appropriate.

Equally, although interviews are a commonly used and valuable method of gathering qualitative information, they need to be the right type of interview. If they are described as highly structured or using closed questions, they are unlikely to give rise to the in-depth answers that would produce qualitative information, and would therefore detract for the study's credibility. Semi-structured or unstructured interviews that use open-ended questions are more likely to give rise to the type of in-depth data required in qualitative research. Interviews may, as Box 7.12 shows, also be face-to-face, conducted by telephone or online, and can be carried out one-to-one, or in a group setting. Each approach has pros and cons. The decisions you have to make in evaluating the quality of a study are:

- whether the approach was congruent with the study's purpose and methodology;
- how far the advantages enhanced study quality;
- how far the disadvantages detracted from the quality of the study;
- what the overall effect of the decisions made was on study quality.

One particular element of all qualitative enquiry is that there should be evidence of the researcher being reflexive (Pilnick and Swift 2010; Zitomer and Goodwin 2014). Qualitative research acknowledges that everyone has opinions, beliefs and experiences that can affect how we interact with others, and interpret and make decisions about data (Pilnick and Swift 2010). Achieving credibility in qualitative research, in terms of the researcher faithfully presenting the participants' views, not their own, therefore requires the researcher to examine their own influence on the study and how it affected the processes of data collection and analysis. Different specific qualitative methodologies handle this issue in different ways. However, in principle, when evaluating a qualitative study you should check whether the researcher acknowledged that their own views and experiences might impact on how data were gathered, analysed or interpreted and explained the steps that they took to address this. These steps could include:

- Using a field journal or diary to make notes about how their previous experiences and input into interactions within the research might have affected the way in which people responded, or how data was interpreted (Whiting 2008; Zitomer and Goodwin 2014).
- Noting their own views, experiences and opinions before undertaking the study, and attempting to 'bracket' or put aside these views so as to avoid them influencing the study (Todres 2005).

- Using respondent validation, where the researchers' interpretations of conversations or events were checked with participants (Houghton *et al.* 2013; Moon *et al.* 2013). Not all studies can achieve this (for example, it may be more challenging to achieve when using group interviews). However, where appropriate, if this is carried out, it enhances the study's credibility.

Pitfall to avoid

Do not assume that the researcher acknowledging that they had views or opinions that might affect the study is a problem in qualitative research. It is how these were dealt with in the research process, not their existence, that matters.

Qualitative studies sometimes use data triangulation, where data gathered from different sources are pieced together to develop a more in-depth insight into the issue under investigation than a single method would achieve (Houghton *et al.* 2013). In ethnography, for instance, prolonged participant observation is often accompanied by some in-depth interviews, to enable the researcher to gain more insight into particular issues that they have noted during their observations. This adds to the study's credibility because a more in-depth and complete picture is gained. However, triangulation only enhances a study's credibility if the methods used are suitable for investigating the matter in question, and enhance understanding of the issue being explored.

7.3.5 Sampling

In qualitative research it is often more appropriate to use non-probability than probability sampling, as the aim is to ensure richness of data and depth of understanding of a contextual issue, not representativeness of a population. Using non-probability sampling offers researchers the opportunity to deliberately select people who are likely to be able to provide in-depth accounts of their experiences, which in turn enhances a study's credibility (Hunt and Lathlean 2015). Examples of approaches to non-probability sampling, and their individual strengths and limitations, are shown in Box 7.6.

Purposive sampling is often seen as particularly useful in qualitative enquiry, because it means that participants can be purposefully sought out who are likely to be able to provide insights into a range of experiences, and to share in-depth information. For example, in a study exploring people's experiences of taking up exercise, purposive sampling might be used in order to select people who had taken up walking, going to the gym, exercise classes and cycling. It might also be used to ensure that the participants included some people who had had positive experiences, some with negative experiences and some who had particular challenges to overcome. This could be a positive attribute of the study, as it would allow the researcher to explore different perspectives in some depth.

It is sometimes useful for qualitative researchers to develop additional selection criteria during the data collection process and to recruit participants to specifically meet these (often using snowballing sampling). In a qualitative study about people's experiences of taking up exercise a researcher might be directed by existing participants to people who could provide them with accounts of particular perspectives that would be of interest. This would increase the depth of understanding of the subject, and also assist the study to avoid being restricted by the researcher's own views or preferences, thus enhancing its credibility.

In order to achieve the in-depth, individual insights required, sample sizes in qualitative research are often small. The concern is not so much how many participants were involved, but whether data were collected in sufficient depth to bring about understanding of the issue of interest (Moon *et al.* 2013). For example, a study which explored the over sixty-fives' experiences of exercising might only include twenty-three participants, because this would enable the researcher to: conduct in-depth interviews with each participant really exploring the nuances of their views and experiences; carefully consider the meaning of every sentence spoken and return to the participants to check whether the way in which what they said had been interpreted was accurate. If a sample of 100 participants was used, this depth of enquiry would be much harder for a single researcher to achieve. Thus, a small sample will often result in a qualitative study achieving credibility, whereas a large sample may detract from the study's quality.

The sample size that will be used in qualitative research is not always pre-specified in the way that is required in quantitative enquiry, because the number of participants needed may depend on when the researcher considers that they have enough depth of information. The point at which this happens (known as data saturation) cannot be pre-specified as it occurs when the researcher notes that no new insights or leads are being offered, and no new theory is being generated (Moon *et al.* 2013; Parahoo 2014). The issue to evaluate in a qualitative study is therefore not the sample size per se.

Instead, it concerns whether the sample would have enabled the study to achieve credibility in terms gaining sufficient depth of understanding of the subject under investigation.

7.3.6 Data analysis

Qualitative data is analysed by the researcher carefully considering the words and meanings that have been shared or observed during data collection, and providing an in-depth interpretation of these (Campos and Turato 2009). The data are usually initially analysed by the researcher reading the information that they have gathered and applying a set of codes or themes to lines or sections that appear to have a particular meaning. Sections of data that appear to have a similar meaning are assigned the same code or theme. These sections are then grouped together so that all the data with a particular code or theme can be seen and understood as a whole. The coded sections are then re-examined and arranged into broader themes or categories (groups of codes or themes that have similar or closely related meanings) (Balls 2009; Campos and Turato 2009).

Exactly how this process is achieved varies, and may be assisted by the use of appropriate computer software. However, qualitative data analysis is essentially achieved by a process of breaking volumes of written data into meaningful chunks and then piecing these together with those deemed to have similar meanings, in order to understand the whole (Campos and Turato 2009). For a study to achieve credibility and dependability, the process of analysing the data should be described in sufficient detail to enable you to judge whether the final outcome is likely to have been a true representation and interpretation of the data gathered (Houghton *et al.* 2013; Moon *et al.* 2013).

The process of analysing qualitative data may be achieved by inductive or deductive means, as outlined in Box 7.13. Whilst inductive processes are perhaps more common, as they closely match the generally inductive nature of qualitative research, what matters in terms of evaluating a study is whether:

- the approach used matches the study design and ethos;
- the process by which codes, themes and categories were developed is clear;
- the links between the study's focus and aims and the codes/themes/categories developed are clear so that the study as a whole is dependable, rigorous and systematic.

> **Box 7.13**
>
> *Inductive vs deductive coding*
>
> *Deductive coding:* topics of interest or codes are chosen before data are analysed.
>
> *Inductive coding:* codes are developed by generating ideas from the data (Bradley *et al.* 2007).

7.3.7 Findings

How a study's findings address its focus and aims should be clear. Unlike quantitative research, the findings from qualitative enquiry should not be based on numerical evaluation, but should describe, explain or draw meaning from large quantities of text in order to address the focus of the research.

Qualitative research reports usually include quotations or excerpts from observations or conversations to substantiate (or lend credibility to) claims to particular findings, or to further illustrate what the researcher meant by a specific point. Although these statements or quotations are usually anonymized, there should be an indication of the range of sources used (for example, by pseudonyms or numbers being allocated to the participants and used to label quotations). There being evidence that the findings include a variety of different perspectives provides some assurance that all the respondents' views were faithfully represented, which enhances the study's credibility (Pilnick and Swift 2010; Moon *et al.* 2013; Houghton *et al.* 2013). For example, if twenty-three people were interviewed about their experiences of engaging in exercise and all the quotes provided were from one or two people, it would bring into question whether the researcher had achieved credibility in terms of representing the experiences of all those involved in the study. On the other hand, if contributions from all twenty-three participants were included at some point in the reported findings, and there was evidence of differing experiences and perspectives on undertaking exercise being represented, the study would seem more credible.

7.3.8 Conclusions and recommendations

The conclusions drawn from any research should address the issue being explored, show that the study aims were met, and be based on what the study's findings showed (Lunenburg and Irby 2008; White 2011). The recommendations made should be derived from the conclusions.

In qualitative enquiry, the conclusions are not intended to be generalizations about what should be done in every situation, but rather should highlight what key issues and considerations the study has unearthed, their importance, and the context in which they were found. In order to achieve this, a qualitative report should provide in-depth information about the context of the study and the nature of participants (Houghton *et al.* 2013; Moon *et al.* 2013). This assists in achieving the criteria of transferability as it enables readers to understand how these factors would have influenced the study findings, and thus to determine whether these are transferable to other particular settings and contexts (Houghton *et al.* 2013; Moon *et al.* 2013).

Whilst there are many broad similarities as to what should be appraised in qualitative and quantitative research, each requires different specific quality criteria to be considered. If the literature that will be included in your review includes mixed methods research, evaluating this will require an understanding of the quality criteria for both qualitative and quantitative research, alongside some additional, specific considerations.

7.4 Appraising mixed methods research

Mixed methods research uses a combination of qualitative and quantitative research methods in a single study (Halcomb *et al.* 2009; Brannan 2015; Turnbull and Lathlean 2015). It is therefore an appropriate approach to use in situations where both quantification and consideration of qualitative aspects of a subject are needed for it to be understood (Halcomb *et al.* 2009; Brannan 2015). The paradigm that underpins mixed methods research is described as pragmatism because, rather than focusing on a particular way of viewing knowledge, the most effective way of exploring the matter in question determines the design and conduct of the research (Turnbull and Lathlean 2015). For instance, a study might aim to ascertain how their experiences of exercising regularly influenced the weight of people over the age of sixty-five. Such a study could beneficially adopt a mixed methods approach, with quantitative methods used to assess participants' weight over a period of time, and qualitative methods to conduct an in-depth exploration of their experiences.

There are not many specific frameworks for evaluating mixed methods studies (MacInnes 2009; Bryman 2014). However, the following areas have been suggested as key considerations in evaluating the quality of mixed methods research:

- Study design: in all research, the study design should match the research question, aim or issue. In mixed methods research, there should be a clear rationale for a mixed methods design being the right approach to use (Venkatesh *et al.* 2013; Bryman 2014; Turnbull and Lathlean 2015).
- The research question or aim: both the qualitative and quantitative elements of a mixed methods study should have clear links with the focus of the study and its aims (Bryman 2014). If any element of the study is not linked to the purpose of the research, its value is questionable, and is likely to detract from the study's logic and system.
- Study design: there are many different ways of designing a mixed methods study, in terms of the weighting, sequence and purpose of the qualitative and quantitative elements. In some cases, it will be appropriate for one method to be the more dominant with the other being complementary or supplementary. In other instances, equal status or weighting may be given to the qualitative and quantitative elements (Turnbull and Lathlean 2015). The design of a mixed methods study, the rationale for this, and how this enables the study's focus to be addressed, should be clear (Bryman 2014).
- Quality of each study component: the quantitative and qualitative components of the study should each be designed and conducted in an appropriate manner (Bryman 2014). In order to assess whether this was achieved, the criteria for evaluating qualitative research should be applied to the qualitative aspects of the study and the criteria for quantitative research to the quantitative elements.
- Key steps in the research process: how the key steps in the research process were conducted should be clear, including how the qualitative and quantitative elements were sequenced and integrated (Bryman 2014). Mixed methods research may be described as sequential (where one method is used after the other), or concurrent (where data are gathered using more than one method at the same time) (Venkatesh *et al.* 2013; Brannan 2015; Turnbull and Lathlean 2015). When evaluating a mixed methods study, a judgement needs to be made concerning how the manner and sequence in which the methods were used contributed to study quality. Box 7.14 shows an example of when a sequential study design might be seen as appropriate in a mixed methods study.
- Integration: there should be a clear sense of a mixed methods study being one unified process of enquiry, rather than two

Box 7.14

Mixed methods study designs

A sequential mixed methods study that aimed to explore whether engaging in exercise assisted people aged over sixty-five to lose weight could begin by using quantitative methods to ascertain whether study participants did or did not lose weight. This could be followed by interviews with a selection of participants who lost weight, gained weight, and whose weight remained the same, to explore in more depth what might have contributed to this. This sequence of data collection would be logical, in that it would be necessary to carry out the quantitative element first in order to select the participants for the qualitative element. It would also contribute to the study being cohesive, as the sampling strategy for the qualitative element would be directly linked to the quantitative element of the study.

separate pieces of research (Venkatesh *et al.* 2013; Bryman 2014; Turnbull and Lathlean 2015). For this to be achieved, the qualitative and quantitative elements of the study need to be integrated in some way, so that the research process as a whole is cohesive (Bryman 2014). Examples of how a mixed methods study might show integration in its sampling and data analysis processes are shown in Boxes 7.15 and 7.16 respectively. This integration of methods to make one unified study is perhaps the key issue in deciding whether a study really meets the criteria required in order for it to be considered as using mixed methods.

Whilst qualitative, quantitative and mixed methods research each have distinct quality indicators, they also have some broad similarities

Box 7.15

Sampling in mixed methods research

- The same sample may be used for both the qualitative and quantitative study elements, for example if a survey is conducted that collects both quantitative and qualitative data.
- There may be two samples, one for the quantitative element of the study and one for the qualitative, but there should be some links or commonalities between the two for the study to be cohesive: for example, one may be drawn from the other or informed by the findings derived from the other.

> ## Box 7.16
>
> *Data analysis in mixed methods research*
>
> Each set of data should be analysed using the right tools for that type of data, but there should also be some connections between the different sets of data, so that the study is cohesive (Venkatesh *et al.* 2013; Bryman 2014; Turnbull and Lathlean 2015).
>
> - Data may be connected by the analysis of one set of data leading to the collection and analysis of another (MacInnes 2009).
> - Qualitative and quantitative data may be collected and analysed together, albeit using different and appropriate methods, so as to gain in-depth understanding of different aspects of a subject (Turnbull and Lathlean 2015).
> - Data transformation may be used so that qualitative data are analysed using quantitative approaches or vice versa (Turnbull and Lathlean 2015). For example, qualitative data may be coded and categorized, but the number of times codes appear may then be quantified. Data transformation creates particular challenges, and the nature of the samples involved, how these fit the analysis processes used and the claims made from such data needs to be carefully considered (Turnbull and Lathlean 2015).

in terms of the requirement for them to demonstrate system, rigour, and to include particular methodological steps. However, depending on the decisions you made about the type of literature to be included in your review, you may also need to appraise information gleaned from audit, evaluation, guidelines, expert opinion and case reports.

7.5 Appraising evaluations and audits

Audit and evaluation have many similarities to research in terms of the processes that they use. The distinction between the three is often described thus: research investigates what should be done; audit investigates whether or not what should be done is being done; and evaluation examines how useful or effective something is or what standard it achieves (National Health Service Health Research Authority 2009, revised 2013). Research may, for instance, involve trialling a potential new treatment. In contrast, audit and evaluation would only involve an intervention or treatment that was already being used, although the outcomes of the audit or evaluation might influence its ongoing use (National Health Service Health Research Authority 2009, revised 2013).

Audit and evaluation should meet similar quality standards to those required in research in so far as they should be conducted using systematic, rigorous and unbiased processes that are appropriate for what they intend to investigate or achieve. They often also use data collection and analysis procedures that are the same as, or very similar to, those seen in research. Because of their similarities to research in terms of process and tools, the criteria used for evaluating research can often be applied to many elements of evaluation and audit.

A key distinction when you are evaluating reports from audit or evaluation activities rather than research is that the processes used to gain permission to carry out audits and evaluations are different from those required for research. Whilst the same ethical principles apply to the conduct of audit, evaluation or research, approval to conduct audits or evaluations is usually obtained through local governance processes rather than ethics committees. In addition, because audit and evaluation are generally designed to examine what is happening in a particular real-world context, with an intervention, treatment or service that is already in place, they do not usually intend to achieve wide generalizability. Box 7.17 gives an example of a distinction between research and evaluation.

7.6 Guidelines, case reports and expert opinion

Guidelines are recommendations, based on the best available evidence, for how particular aspects of care should be provided (National Institute for Health and Care Excellence 2014). The quality of a guideline depends on the information that has been used to inform its development and the manner in which that information has been interpreted and presented. A guideline that is based on a rigorous and systematic analysis of all the available evidence is likely to itself be high-quality evidence. However, if a guideline does not indicate the basis for its recommendations it is difficult to judge its quality. When you are appraising a guideline, you should therefore examine the evidence on which its recommendations are based, and whether the recommendations made are commensurate with the quality and strength of that evidence. A tool that has been developed to assist in appraising practice guidelines is the AGREE II tool (Brouwers et al. 2010), available at www.agreetrust.org/agree-ii/.

Box 7.17

Research and evaluation

Research:
At present, there is no particular exercise programme recommended for people aged over sixty-five who need to lose weight. Joe plans to set up a research study in which people over 65 years of age who are overweight and who agree to participate are randomly allocated to either:

• receive specific advice on undertaking exercise and the opportunity to participate in exercise classes;

or

• be given the usual advice on weight loss.

The weight changes in each group will then be compared. Joe hopes to design a study that allows generalization to the population of people aged over sixty-five.

Evaluation:
Joe has, for the last year, been offering specific advice, guidance and the opportunity to attend exercise classes to people aged over sixty-five who are overweight. He now wants to evaluate the effectiveness of this service, by checking whether or not those who attended the classes have lost weight. Joe's intention is to evaluate whether this particular service is proving effective, in the context in which he works.

Case reports usually report a case or cases of a particular condition, disorder, disease or situation, describe and analyse what happened in that case, and should ideally offer reasoned and critically considered explanations for it. However, they do not generally adopt as systematic or rigorous a process to their enquiry as is required in research (Gopikrishna 2010). In addition, because they only intend to report on a small number of cases (often one), they do not claim any degree of generalizability. When you evaluate a case report, key issues to consider are whether:

• the report presents a logical, well-thought-out discussion;
• different possible reasons for the outcomes seen are discussed critically;
• there is any evidence of bias;
• the claims made are commensurate with the preceding discussion.

Expert opinion constitutes the opinion of an expert or experts in a particular field of work. Although this can be a valuable source of information, the basis for claims to expertise varies, and thus the inherent quality of expert opinion is also variable. Expert opinion is not usually considered to be as strong a form of evidence as research, because the views of experts may not be a result of the systematic approach to enquiry that is demanded in research (Gopikrishna 2010). Consensus expert opinion is generally seen as preferable to an individual's view, because it is less likely to be subjective. Often case reports and expert opinion are combined, as an expert in the field will provide a case report, in which they use their expertise to analyse the key issues involved in that case.

When you are evaluating the quality of a report that is based on expert opinion, some of the things that you should consider are:

- What is the basis of the person's claim to expertise?
- Is their argument logical and supported by evidence?
- Is their argument well balanced, showing analysis of their opinions, and explaining how these were reached?

The process of appraising every piece of evidence that will form a part of your literature review, using criteria appropriate for the type of literature in question, enables you to make judgements about their quality. This information will, as Chapter 8 describes, subsequently be used to synthesize your findings from each paper into a composite whole. To this end, you should record your observations as you evaluate each paper.

7.7 Recording evaluative data

As you appraise each piece of literature that you have selected for review, you should record the key points that you have observed about it. This will provide a clear audit trail of your activities, assist you to recall the decisions that you made accurately, and thereby aid you in the task of synthesizing the evidence as a whole, and making recommendations from it. The information that you record should include:

- the nature of the evidence;
- the findings related to the review question;
- the quality of the evidence (and how you reached the decisions you did about this);
- the strength of the evidence (and how you determined this).

Any studies that are of such poor quality that they should be disregarded may be excluded from the synthesis of the findings described in Chapter 8. However, your report should clarify that these findings have been excluded, and why this decision was made, including what the quality cut-off point was and why this point was selected (Hemingway and Brereton 2009; Aveyard 2014: 87–8). This will enable your reader to understand the decisions that you made, why you made them, and assure them that any data omitted from the synthesis of evidence were excluded on the basis of quality, not bias.

Pitfall to avoid

Do not forget to record your decisions about the nature and quality of each paper that you appraise in a way that will make sense to you later on, remind you of your key decisions and why they were made.

Summary

All the evidence that you have gathered for your literature review should be individually appraised, using criteria that are appropriate for the type of evidence in question. You may decide to use an existing tool or tools to assist you in this; however, the key issue is that the processes that you follow to make decisions about the quality of each paper should be rigorous, systematic, unbiased and transparent. As you appraise the individual papers you should make comprehensive notes about the decisions that you make. This will add to the rigour and system of your study by providing clear and recorded evidence of how you made the decisions that you did. It will also enable you to recall these decisions as you synthesize the evidence from across sources.

Terminology

Audit: investigates whether or not what should be done is being done (NHS Health Research Authority 2009, revised 2013).

Case reports: reports of a case or cases of a particular condition, disorder, disease or situation that describe and analyse what happened in that case, and offer reasoned and critically considered explanations for it.

Evaluation studies: studies that examine how useful or effective something is, or what standard it achieves (NHS Health Research Authority 2009, revised 2013).

Expert opinion: the opinion of an expert or experts in a particular field of practice.

Guidelines: recommendations based on the best available evidence regarding how particular aspects of care should be provided (National Institute for Health and Care Excellence 2014).

Mixed methods research: (pragmatic paradigm) research that uses a combination of qualitative and quantitative methods in a single study.

Qualitative research: (interpretivist or naturalistic research) research that aims to achieve in-depth understanding by gaining insight into individual, subjective and contextual factors that influence and affect people and situations.

Quantitative research: (positivist research) research that views truth as objective, not dependent on context or interpretation.

Key points:

- In order to identify the composite evidence on the subject being reviewed, the findings from the evaluation of the individual papers included in that review need to be synthesized.
- Evidence can be synthesized using a variety of methods, including meta-analysis, meta-synthesis and mixed methods synthesis.
- In literature review methodology, where the types of evidence included are often heterogeneous, narrative synthesis is commonly the most appropriate approach to use.

The intention of conducting a study that uses literature review methodology is to identify what the current evidence about a particular subject is. Therefore, whilst evaluating each individual paper that is included in your study (as described in Chapter 7) is a vital stage in the literature review process, it is not the end point. If a literature review does not go beyond discussing the findings, strengths and limitations of each individual piece of evidence its only real contribution to the body of knowledge is to provide an evaluation of individual papers. In order to identify the composite evidence on a subject, the findings from across all the individual papers that have been appraised need to be synthesized. By synthesizing the findings from across sources a literature review adds to the current evidence by establishing what is and is not already known about the subject in question, and demonstrating the overall consistency and strength of the existing evidence. This synthesis should demonstrate:

- what each individual piece of evidence claims;
- the quality and strength of each piece of evidence;
- how each piece of evidence compares with the other evidence on the subject;
- why similarities and differences in the evidence from different sources may exist;

- any gaps in the evidence;
- what the composite existing evidence on the subject therefore is.

All the stages involved in a study that uses literature review methodology should be systematic and rigorous, and the process of synthesizing the findings from across sources is no exception to this rule (Rodgers *et al.* 2009). There is a range of established methods that can be used to perform such syntheses, including meta-analysis, meta-synthesis, mixed methods synthesis and narrative synthesis. If you are using literature review methodology rather than carrying out a systematic review, it is likely that you will use a form of narrative synthesis, as described later in this chapter, in your review. It is, nonetheless, useful to understand the other options that exist, so that you are aware of the principles that underpin them, and understand why they are, or are not, appropriate for your study. In addition, you may have included systematic reviews that use meta-analysis, meta-synthesis or mixed methods synthesis in the literature that you have used. Knowing about the ways in which data may have been synthesized in such reviews should assist you to understand what was, and was not, done and whether this was appropriate for the study in question.

8.1 Meta-analysis

Meta-analysis refers to a range of statistical processes that can be used to synthesize the findings from particular types of quantitative research. By combining the data from across two or more studies, meta-analysis effectively increases the sample size being analysed. This means that the results gleaned from the meta-analysis can be more certain and precise than those from each individual study could be (Haidich 2010). For instance, a review of noise levels in intensive care units (ICUs) might include five individual studies that measured the noise level at night on ICUs. The first might measure noise levels over forty days, the second over twenty days, and the other three over thirty days each. Combining the results from across all five studies using meta-analysis would effectively give a sample of 150 days, rather than twenty, thirty, or forty days. This would allow more precise and generalizable statistical results regarding noise levels on ICUs to be determined than would be possible in each individual study.

Although meta-analysis uses numerical data, it cannot be used for every type of quantitative data. It was at one time generally only used to pool data from randomized controlled trials. However, it is now thought that non-randomized data can also be used for meta-analysis, although there is debate as to how such data should be dealt with, and the quality of the resultant findings (Crombie and Davies 2009; Haidich 2010; Onitilo 2014). By combining the data from across studies, meta-analysis effectively considers all the data sets as one. Therefore, the greater the similarity in the study design and outcomes being measured across all the included studies, the more precise the analysis can be (Crombie and Davies 2009; Haidich 2010; Onitilo 2014). As a result, the more closely matched the studies included in a meta-analysis are, the more accurate the findings are, in principle, likely to be. In the example of measuring noise levels in ICUs, if data were pooled from five studies in which noise was measured in the same way, from comparable locations (albeit on different ICUs), at the same times, it would be able to be more accurately viewed as one set of data than if noise was measured in different ways, from disparate locations within the ICUs, and at different times.

Meta-analysis is often used in systematic reviews of the effectiveness of interventions. However, for many studies that use literature review methodology, and that do not aim or claim to comply with the requirements of a systematic review, attempting to undertake a meta-analysis is not appropriate. Often, the studies included in a literature review will not be similar enough in terms of aims and design for a meta-analysis to be a viable choice. If the study you are undertaking does not meet the criteria for performing a meta-analysis you should not undertake one. In addition, if you do not have the resources in terms of statistical knowledge, software and backup to carry out a rigorous, systematic and accurate meta-analysis, then you should not select this option.

Meta-analysis deals with quantitative data, but there are broadly equivalent processes that can be used to synthesize qualitative data. These are often collectively referred to as meta-synthesis.

Pitfall to avoid

Attempting to conduct a meta-analysis will not, of itself, improve the quality of your review. A meta-analysis only adds to the quality of a study if it is appropriate to conduct one, and you have the necessary resources and skills to do so.

8.2 Meta-synthesis

'Meta-synthesis' is an umbrella term that can be used to describe a variety of processes of synthesizing data from more than one qualitative study in order to develop, enlarge or broaden understanding of the issue being explored (Egerod *et al.* 2015). Because meta-synthesis deals with qualitative rather than quantitative data, it does not usually aim to increase the precision of measurement or the generalizability of the findings from across studies by increasing the sample size. Instead, by comparing, contrasting and analysing the perspectives gained from different studies, it aims to produce a richer, deeper and more insightful understanding of the topic of interest (Saini and Shlonsky 2012).

In the same way that meta-analysis can use a number of different specific statistical tests, there are several techniques that can be used to carry out a meta-synthesis, depending on the types of study included and the aim of the synthesis. These approaches include: meta-ethnography, critical interpretative synthesis, meta-narrative, and thematic synthesis (Barnett-Page and Thomas 2009; Egerod *et al.* 2015). The processes used, however, all essentially involve reviewing and analysing the themes, findings or conclusions that were developed in individual studies, considering in-depth their meaning compared to those in other studies, and forming these into a coherent whole (Saini and Shlonsky 2012). Achieving this requires the reviewer to identify ideas, codes, themes or categories within the individual studies, then to compare and develop these across sources so as to produce an in-depth analysis of the data from all the included studies.

A qualitative meta-synthesis of patients' experience of noise on ICUs might, for instance, use the evidence from six different qualitative studies. By reviewing the data gathered in these studies the synthesis could:

- develop additional themes, codes or categories to those developed in the original studies;
- identify how the themes, codes, categories or insights seen in one study might apply to the data from the other studies;
- gain a more in-depth understanding of the themes, codes or categories that already exist by identifying additional nuances in the data when the studies are viewed as a whole.

The synthesis of the findings from across studies might also deepen understanding of the topic of interest by increasing the breadth of the experiences reported, and including in the synthesis perspectives that were unique to each study.

When you are undertaking a study that uses literature review methodology, rather than a systematic review, the information that you have gathered may not be based on studies whose focus and design are sufficiently similar to use meta-synthesis. In addition, the resources available to you may mean that you cannot use this approach. For example, meta-synthesis, whilst not requiring statistical expertise, often requires more than one reviewer (to ensure that the depth of the coding processes required is achieved, and biases are minimized). As with meta-analysis, if the data or resources that you have are not commensurate with conducting a good quality meta-synthesis, you should not attempt to use this approach.

Meta-analysis and meta-synthesis both deal with studies from within particular research paradigms. However, in some cases it is useful to synthesize the findings from a mix of qualitative and quantitative studies. In this case, mixed methods synthesis can be a useful approach to use.

> **Pitfall to avoid**
>
> Attempting to undertake a meta-synthesis will not necessarily enhance the quality of your review. It is better to carry out a synthesis that is appropriate for the aim, scope and resources of your review, and to do that well, than to attempt something that will not work.

8.3 Mixed methods synthesis

As Chapter 7 discussed, mixed methods research (where a single study includes both qualitative and quantitative approaches to data collection and analysis) is becoming well established as a valuable approach to enquiry (Halcomb *et al.* 2009; Brannan 2015; Turnbull and Lathlean 2015). Mixed methods synthesis, wherein the findings from qualitative and quantitative research are synthesized into one overall evidence base, is similarly increasingly being recognized as a useful approach (Hemingway and Brereton 2009).

Mixed methods synthesis employs appropriate methods to synthesize the findings from qualitative and quantitative research on a given subject. How this is achieved varies, depending on the aim of the synthesis, and the research that is included in it. However, as with mixed methods research, mixed methods synthesis differs from two separate syntheses that explore related issues. In order to merit the term 'mixed methods', the synthesis has to assimilate the synthesized findings from the qualitative and quantitative sources in some way. As a result, the findings must present the evidence from across all the studies as one integrated whole, rather than as two separate sets of data.

A mixed methods synthesis concerning noise in ICUs might include a meta-analysis of six studies that measured noise levels on

ICUs. The qualitative element might comprise of a meta-synthesis of five studies concerning people's perceptions of noise whilst they were cared for on an ICU. A link might then be made between the two sets of synthesized data by identifying whether the loudest, most frequent or disruptive noise as shown in the meta-analysis matched what the meta-synthesis showed patients to consider the most disturbing. If this was not the case, the reasons for any differences could be explored. Thus, both data sets would be used to inform one another, and to enable the reviewer to develop a critical discussion of the evidence base as a whole. This type of link between the qualitative and quantitative data would enable the synthesis to claim the term 'mixed methods'.

Whilst mixed methods synthesis uses data from both qualitative and quantitative research, it still focuses on using techniques such as meta-analysis and meta-synthesis to interpret and analyse data. Therefore, a mixed methods synthesis will also often fall outside the realms of a study that uses literature review methodology. In such studies, the most appropriate approach to use is often a form a narrative synthesis.

8.4 Narrative approaches to synthesis

Studies that use literature review methodology often draw on information that is too diverse in nature to use meta-analysis or meta-synthesis. In addition, these procedures often require more than one reviewer, and, in the case of meta-analysis, access to specific statistical expertise and software, which can render them unsuitable for studies which lack the funding to procure such resources. It is often therefore most appropriate for studies that use literature review methodology to adopt a form of narrative synthesis to develop a composite picture of the evidence from across studies (Ryan 2013).

If, for instance, you were conducting a literature review on the subject of how patients experience noise in the ICU, you might find ten relevant papers comprising:

- four quantitative studies (one involving the measurement of noise levels on ICUs, two cross-sectional surveys of patients' recollections of noise on ICUs using different questionnaires, and one cross-sectional survey of nurses' views on how noise affects patients on ICUs);
- four qualitative studies that explore patients' recollections of noise on the ICU;

- an evaluation of an innovation aimed at reducing noise on an ICU that explores patients' perspectives using a post discharge questionnaire;
- One paper, written by an expert in the field, on the physiological effects of noise on patients on ICUs.

The quantitative papers include different study designs, and the cross-sectional surveys, despite having the same basic study design, do not use the same (or very similar) questionnaires. They also include one study that obtained data from a different population group from the others. Therefore, even if it were feasible in terms of resources and expertise, a meta-analysis would not be an appropriate way to synthesize the findings from these papers. The qualitative papers might be amenable to a meta-synthesis, but this would mean excluding all the other papers. The final two papers do not contain data derived from research, and therefore do not fit the requirements for a meta-analysis or meta-synthesis. Overall, therefore, meta-analysis, meta-synthesis or mixed methods synthesis would not be appropriate approaches to adopt to synthesize the findings from these studies. A narrative synthesis would be a better approach to take. This would be achievable, and could be performed in a logical, rigorous and systematic way. In contrast, attempting to use the other approaches would result in a flawed study whose methodology and method lacked the requisite system and rigour.

The term 'narrative synthesis' describes a range of approaches to synthesizing data from across sources (Snilstveit *et al.* 2012). Because of the range of approaches that it encompasses, narrative synthesis can be used to address many different types of review questions and aims, and can draw on a variety of sources of data. This flexibility makes it a very useful option for literature review methodology, in which many variations in study question, aim, design and included literature exist. However, it also means that there is no absolute consensus about the specific steps and processes that should be involved in a narrative synthesis (Rodgers *et al.* 2009). For instance, a narrative synthesis designed to collate the findings from seven cross-sectional surveys would need to use a very different approach to one synthesizing the findings from a variety of quantitative, qualitative and mixed methods studies. However, the specific processes adopted in any synthesis should be justified, rigorous, systematic, transparent and unbiased (Snilstveit *et al.* 2012; Ryan 2013). To this end, the procedures that you use, and why you select these, should be detailed in your study methodology.

Whilst the exact processes that should be followed in a narrative synthesis vary, the synthesis should provide a logical, analytical and comprehensive story (or narrative) of the current best evidence (Rodgers *et al.* 2009; Roberts and Bailey 2011). In order to achieve this, there are four steps that should usually form the basis for most narrative syntheses. These are:

- determining the themes or categories into which data will be placed;
- summarizing the individual papers;
- synthesizing the data from across all the papers included in the review;
- critically reviewing the synthesis.

(Ryan 2013)

8.4.1 Determining the themes or categories into which data will be placed

Narrative synthesis uses non-statistical approaches to identifying and synthesizing the findings from all the papers that are included in a review (Ryan 2013). This is usually achieved by developing themes, codes or categories into which the information from the different sources that you have can be allocated. The information from each paper that has been allocated to a particular theme, code or category is then placed together so that each theme, code or category can be considered as a whole. Exactly how you develop these codes, themes or categories will depend on the nature of your study, its question and aims, and the papers that are included.

You may decide to develop the codes, categories or themes that you will use deductively. If, as described by Le Boiutelier *et al.* (2015), your study is designed to test a particular theory, you will probably have decided on some of the key comparisons that you wish to make before undertaking the synthesis. These will then become some of your themes, codes or categories. If you are carrying out a narrative synthesis of noise in ICUs, based on the theory that nurses' perspectives on noise differs from patients' perspectives, one theme or code would probably be 'nurses' views', and one 'patients' views'.

Your study aims may also provide you with deductive codes that you want to use or develop. For example, if your study question was: 'Do nurses' and patients' perspectives on noise on ICUs differ?' your aims might include:

- To identify whether nurses perceive daytime noise differently from patients.

- To ascertain whether nurses perceive night-time noise differently from patients.
- To explore the priority that nurses give to reducing noise.
- To examine the priority that patients believe reducing noise should be allotted.

In this case, you would probably expect to have codes, themes or categories related to noise at night from nurses' perspectives, noise during the day from nurses' perspectives, noise at night from patients' perspectives, noise during the day from patients' perspectives, nurses' views on the priority of noise reduction, and patients' views on the priority of noise reduction.

In other circumstances, depending on your study question and aims, it may be more appropriate to develop the codes, themes or categories that you will use inductively. In this case, these will be developed as you read and evaluate the papers that are included in your study, for example by considering what the theories, explanations or key findings in the papers are (Ryan 2013). There are also instances where it is appropriate to develop the themes for a narrative review by using a combination of deductive and inductive approaches. For instance, you may begin by using deductive coding based on a pre-specified theory, your study question and aims. However, as you analyse each paper, these codes may be augmented by an inductive approach that enables you to identify additional new codes, gain new insights and explore unexpected findings (Le Boiutelier et al. 2015).

As well as codes, themes or categories that relate to the theories, insights, findings and conclusions in the papers, you may also decide to include categories, codes or themes related to:

- the characteristics of the studies (for example, you might have categories devoted to qualitative evidence, quantitative evidence, randomized controlled trials, mixed methods studies, case reports, or papers based on expert opinion) (Ryan 2013);
- the characteristics of participants (Ryan 2013) (for example, evidence about people who were on ICU long term compared to those who only had a very short stay; people who underwent planned admission to ICU compared to those who were admitted as an emergency).

The way in which you develop the codes, themes or categories for your synthesis must be rigorous, systematic and appropriate for what you are trying to achieve. For instance, you may decide to use a combination of inductive and deductive coding. If you do so, as you inductively develop new codes, themes or categories during the process of data analysis, you will need to recheck the papers that you had analysed before developing these to ensure that you have not missed any relevant data. It is also very common for the codes, themes or categories that you initially develop to be further refined during the process of data synthesis (Roberts and Bailey 2011). If this is the case, as you refine your thinking, you should revisit previously analysed papers to ensure that the way in which you have allocated data is congruent with these new insights. It is important to keep a record of the decisions that you make about how and why you develop each code, theme or category and what each one means. This ensures that what you do is transparent, allows you to revisit these decisions later on, review them, and to check that you applied the codes, themes or categories consistently and systematically to every part of your data. These decisions, and the processes that you followed to ensure that the analysis process was rigorous, systematic and unbiased, should be documented in your study methodology.

Pitfall to avoid

Do not assume that you will remember all the decisions that you made as you analysed the literature. Instead, make notes about every stage of the process, and your decisions, as you go.

Having decided on how you will develop and use the codes, themes or categories for your synthesis, the next step in the process of narrative synthesis is to apply these decisions to the papers that you have reviewed. To achieve this, you should note the parts (lines, sentences or whole sections) of each paper that could be described by using each code, theme or category. If you are developing the themes or codes inductively the reading and coding of papers and their development will occur simultaneously.

As you code the papers, you should record the relevant extracts from each one, so that these can be grouped and collated after you have completed reading and analysing all the literature that you have collected (Le Boiutelier et al. 2015). How you make these extracts and record them will depend on how you prefer to work, but what needs to be achieved is a system by which you can place all the identically themed, coded or categorized extracts from the different papers into one group.

There is no single best way of developing the categories for a narrative synthesis that you must adhere to. The approach you use should be led by your study question and aim, and the type of literature included in your review.

Many people also find it useful to devise a table or chart which outlines:

- the codes, themes or categories that were developed;
- when and how they were developed;
- which studies contributed to each one.

This provides a quick reference guide for yourself and your reader about the processes followed, and shows evidence of system and rigour in your analysis.

8.4.2 Summarizing the individual papers that are included in the review

The second step in the process of narrative synthesis is to develop a brief description of each of the papers that have been included in your review, based around the findings from your analysis of the individual papers (as described in Chapter 7) (Ryan 2013). This description should summarize the key features for each paper, such as:

- the type of evidence involved;
- the research question, aim or issue being explored;
- the study design (where appropriate);
- the population dealt with in the paper;
- the methods used (where appropriate);
- the key findings;
- the conclusions and recommendations.
- the key strengths and limitations of the paper.

(Ryan 2013)

It is usually useful to arrange these summaries so that you describe the key features of each paper in the same order, to make it easy for your reader to see the similarities and differences between them (Aveyard 2014: 144–50). Where your synthesis includes more than one study design or type of evidence, grouping papers of similar kinds together makes your report logical and user-friendly, for example by presenting the summaries of all the quantitative studies first, then all the qualitative studies, followed by those derived from other forms of evidence. Many people find it helpful to accompany this description of the studies with a table that outlines their key features.

This stage of the process of narrative synthesis should, then, provide a clear, detailed but concise summary of each paper that has been included in the review. This demonstrates that you conducted your evaluation of the individual studies in a rigorous and systematic fashion, and have a good understanding of them. However, whilst this is a vital part of the study findings, to achieve a narrative synthesis, the analysis process needs to go beyond summarizing, discussing and analysing the main features of each paper (Ryan 2013). It needs to be followed by the integration of the outcomes of the first two stages outlined above. To achieve this, a combined narrative of the codes, categories or themes that have been developed, and the key aspects of each paper, is created in order to form a synthesis of the evidence derived from the studies as a whole. Exactly how you carry out this next stage will depend on the range of papers that you have, how you developed your codes, categories and themes, and what they are.

8.4.3 Synthesizing the data from across all the papers included in the review

Having appraised each individual paper as described in Chapter 7, and developed and applied appropriate codes, themes or categories to describe the content of the papers, this information needs to be developed into a coherent whole (Ryan 2013). This process often requires the information from the individual papers to be transformed so that it is all in a format that is amenable to the approach to synthesis that you are using. If you have the following, you will need to decide how you will transform the information contained in each type of study so that you can present a narrative of the whole (Ryan 2013):

- three studies measuring levels of noise on ICUs;
- two cross-sectional surveys of patients' experiences of noise on ICUs;
- three qualitative studies of patients' experiences on noise on ICUs.

This transformation of data should not in any way alter the meaning of the information, but is rather intended to frame it in terminology that enables it to be used to tell the story of what you found across all the literature included in your review. It is also necessary so that your narrative can meaningfully and analytically compare and contrast the findings from different papers, rather than simply describing each one in turn.

In the example given, it might be essential to retain the numerical measures obtained in the first study. However, your narrative of these numbers would explain and explore which of these measurements were considered commensurate with a high level of noise, what was seen as lower, etc. This information would also be entwined with the findings from other studies, so that your narrative explored, for instance, whether patients reported the greatest disturbance from events that were recorded as being very noisy. It might also discuss how you compared what one study termed a high level of noise and how another study described this.

Exactly how you structure your synthesis will depend on what has been most important in your findings, what codes, themes or categories you have developed, and what will provide a logical narrative for your reader. Ryan (2013) suggests that papers of different types, or studies with different designs, should be discussed in separate sections of the synthesis, as these variations will result in different methodological strengths and weaknesses, which will be better discussed as groups. In your synthesis of the findings you may therefore wish to have sections devoted to discussing the findings from particular types of evidence. For example, if your review included randomized controlled trials (RCTs) and case control studies, your synthesis could include a section on the data from RCTs, and a section related to the case control studies (Ryan 2013).

Whether or not you can adopt this approach will, however, depend on the variety of studies that are included in your review. If, for instance, you have seven papers, all derived from different types of evidence, such a structure will not be achievable. You might, in this instance, choose to have a section of your synthesis that concerns methodological issues that have influenced the overall evidence base of the study. This could include an analysis of the relevant similarities and differences in design, population, and methods between the studies that you have included, exploring why these are important, and how they affect the overall evidence base (Ryan 2013).

In other cases, the type of evidence included in your review and the key issues that you have identified in your analysis of the individual studies may render it most appropriate to comment on methodological issues within sections devoted to particular findings. For instance, you might decide that it is appropriate to have a section of your narrative synthesis entitled: 'Patients' perspectives on noise at night' in which you discuss all the findings related to noise at night on ICUs from patients' perspectives, regardless of the study design involved. Within this section, you would then explore not just the findings regarding this aspect of noise on the ICU, but how different study designs contributed to the particular perspectives identified, and to the strengths and limitations of the overall evidence base. No one approach to presenting the findings in a narrative synthesis is always right or wrong. What is critical is that your decisions match the data that you have, and that your reader can follow your narrative and see the logic behind how it is presented.

Having conducted this preliminary synthesis, decided what will go where in your narrative, and how your arguments will develop, an analysis of the narrative within each category needs to be developed. Within the themes, codes or categories that you have developed the evidence from different sources may corroborate each other (for example, the measured noise levels in one study may correspond very well with events that patients in another study reported as particularly disturbing), or they may show different findings (the events which were recorded as particularly noisy may not be those that most disturbed patients). Your task as you synthesize the findings is to faithfully represent the range and depth of data that you encounter. You are not required to try to demonstrate a whole in which there is agreement between studies. Rather, it is your responsibility to show where disconfirming evidence exists as well as where there is agreement, and to explore possible reasons for this.

Whether you place differing perspectives in the same or separate sections of your synthesis will depend on how you have developed and structured your codes, themes and categories, and the overall content of your synthesis. However, the synthesis as a whole must demonstrate that you explored, rather than tried to reduce or ignore, differing viewpoints. There may, of course, be some instances where no disconfirming views are seen across all the evidence, and where the studies' findings are all congruent with one another. In such situations, it is useful to identify this in your synthesis, so that it is clear to your reader that you have presented the whole story of the data from across studies, and that disconfirming data have not been omitted.

Pitfall to avoid

Do not think that you need to show that there is conformity of evidence across the literature that is included in your review. Your task is to show the true range of evidence and to explore the possible reasons for differences and similarities between the findings from different studies.

The synthesis of the findings in your study should, then, include a discussion of the commonalities and distinctions between the evidence included in your review, but also why these might exist. However, as a prelude to this in-depth analysis, vote counting can be used to give an overall impression of the similarities and differences between the papers (Ryan 2013; Le Boiutelier *et al.* 2015). This involves performing a simple count to identify the number of papers showing a particular outcome or viewpoint compared with those showing the opposing view, a neutral view, or not discussing the issue at all. If you were synthesizing the findings from seven studies that explored patients' experiences of noise on the ICU, and had noise from machinery as a theme, you might use vote counting to provide a basic overview of how many studies indicated that noise from machinery was disruptive. This process does not, however, take into account the quality of the studies, or why particular outcomes or views gained a vote. Thus, as Ryan (2013) states, it is a perfectly acceptable introductory statement to a discussion of particular findings, but needs to be followed by a more in-depth analysis of these.

This exploration and analysis includes critically considering the findings from each paper, comparing the findings between each one, and the possible reasons for the differences and similarities in these. This might include whether the methodologies, methods, populations of the studies, overall quality of the studies, biases and confounders might account for any differences found (Le Boiutelier *et al.* 2015). Equally, in some instances, there may be no clear reason for any differences in the findings between studies, and where this is the case your narrative should outline what possible causes you considered, and how you ruled these out.

Because your aim is to provide an in-depth synthesis of the findings from across the papers that you have included, you need to look beyond the obvious in your exploration. The variations in the questions, aims, methodologies and designs of the studies included in your review are likely to mean that the links between, and reasons for, any apparent differences between findings may not be immediately obvious (Ryan 2013). It is therefore worth devoting considerable time to reading, exploring, re-exploring and critically thinking about the data included in each code, theme or category. This will assist you in moving the process beyond being a superficial description to achieving the required in-depth exploration of your data. It will also enable you to demonstrate that you have considered the possible explanations for what you have found in a logical and systematic way, and carefully weighed up the nature and strength of the evidence that exists within each theme, code or category (Ryan 2013; Rodgers *et al.* 2009).

Pitfall to avoid

Do not accept obvious or superficial reasons for any differences between the findings from the studies included in your review. Take time to consider, reconsider and reflect on the range of possibilities that exist.

At the end of this stage of the process of narrative synthesis you should have developed a logical, and systematic, synthesis of the findings from across the papers that constitute your study data. However, the final step of your narrative synthesis is to revisit your review, check its quality, and identify the strengths and limitations of what you have been able to achieve.

8.4.4 Critically reviewing the synthesis

To ensure that you are making a suitable claim concerning the strength of the evidence that you are presenting, you should evaluate the robustness of the synthesis that you have conducted (Ryan 2013; Le Boiutelier *et al.* 2015). To achieve this, you should revisit each of the stages of your synthesis and critically reflect on (Ryan 2013):

- the strengths and limitations of the methods that you have used at each point;
- why you made the decisions that you did;
- how these decisions have contributed to the quality of the study as a whole.

This may enable you to make adjustments to any processes that, on reflection, could be improved and that can be altered without detracting from the rigour, system and robustness of the study. For example, as you revisit your work you may realize that a particular issue affected the quality of some of the studies, but that you have not developed a theme about this or alluded to it in your discussion. This information could then be added, either to your discussion of an existing theme, or as a further inductively developed theme, and its development noted in your log of how the themes used in the review were developed.

Whilst possible improvements in your work may come to your attention as you perform your evaluation, most studies have some limitations that are outside your control and cannot be altered. These should be included in a discussion of the overall strengths and limitations of the review. Including a discussion of known weaknesses in the synthesis that you have performed demonstrates to your reader that your study is transparent, and does not seek to conceal its limitations. Weighing up the strengths and limitations of the synthesis also informs the strength of your conclusions, and your recommendations for future reviews and research (Ryan 2013).

Your discussion of the strengths and limitations of your synthesis may include whether the papers that you included were able to sufficiently address the review question and aims. Any parts of the study question or aims that could not be addressed should be highlighted, and the reasons for this outlined. In some cases, despite gathering all the available literature on a subject, you may have found that none of the papers sufficiently addressed one particular aim of your review. In this instance, that aim may be unmet, for reasons outside your control. Acknowledging this, and why the aim remains unmet, is an important part of demonstrating that your review followed a systematic process (in so far as the aim is accounted for, and not seen to be forgotten). It is also an important finding, as it is likely to suggest that primary research, focused on the aim in question, would be beneficial.

A section on any potential biases in the review process that might have affected the findings is also useful to include. This should include an evaluation of the assumptions made throughout the review process, and how these were managed when analysing the data (Ryan 2013).

Having conducted these four steps, you will be ready to present your synthesis as a narrative report.

8.5 Presenting synthesized data in a narrative report

It is often useful to begin the presentation of the synthesized evidence by providing an overview of the general points that you discovered: for example, how many papers were included in the review; how many were of each particular type of evidence; the location of the studies; years of publication; and why each of these issues were important.

This introductory paragraph will usually be followed by a brief summary of each paper, often accompanied by a table demonstrating the key points related to each one. The codes, categories or themes that were used and how these were developed can then be presented (or the other way around, depending on which gives a more logical flow to your writing). This is usually followed by the in-depth discussion of each code, theme or category that will form the body of your synthesis of the findings. In order to give structure and logic to your report it is often sensible to use each theme, code or category as a subheading, and to define it, before entering into your exploration of the findings within it.

Finally, you may decide to include in the synthesis of the findings what the key strengths and limitations of your own review are. Some people prefer to leave exploring these to a later part of their study, such as the discussion (which is discussed in Chapter 9), or to have a specific section for them. However, they should be included somewhere before the stage at which you make your conclusions, and, because these affect the nature of your synthesized evidence, many people see this as a logical place to locate them.

This part of the report on your review of the literature should, therefore, convey to your reader what the composite evidence related to your study question and aims is. It should do this analytically, systematically and logically, and should answer the review question or questions clearly. The answer to these questions may be anything: it may be that you are able to unequivocally provide a precise answer to the question you posed. It may equally be that at present the evidence on the subject is not conclusive, and more research (and possibly more research of a particular type) is needed. However, for the review as a whole to be rigorous and systematic, the synthesis of the findings should address the study question and demonstrate that the study aims have been met.

Summary

There are a variety of methods of synthesizing the findings from more than one study, including meta-analysis, meta-synthesis, mixed methods synthesis and narrative synthesis. Most studies that use literature review methodology will, however, use a form of narrative synthesis. The exact processes involved in this type of synthesis vary, depending on the papers included in the study in question. In general, though, narrative synthesis follows four distinct stages: developing themes or categories, summarizing individual papers, synthesizing the themes or categories from across papers, and finally reviewing the quality of the process of synthesis (Ryan 2013). These steps should be used to enable you to compare and contrast the evidence from across all the sources used in your review, so as to critically evaluate the composite best evidence across the literature as a whole.

Terminology

Deductive coding: codes are chosen before data are analysed.

Inductive coding: codes are developed by generating ideas from the data (Bradley *et al.* 2007).

Meta-analysis: statistical processes used to synthesize the findings from more than one quantitative study.

Meta-synthesis: processes used to synthesize data from more than one qualitative study.

Mixed methods synthesis: a process that synthesizes the findings from qualitative and quantitative research on a given subject.

Narrative synthesis: A narrative approach to summarizing and synthesizing the evidence on a given subject.

Key points:

- The discussion section of a study that uses literature review methodology should interrogate the findings from the review, and integrate these with the more general literature related to the subject.
- The discussion should be focused on the findings from the review, but should interpret, develop and explore these in greater depth.
- This part of the review should bring the key issues from the study together so as to enable you to draw conclusions and make recommendations.

The main purpose of the discussion section of a literature review is to pull together all the threads of the study (Murray 2011). By this stage, the rationale for the review, how it was conducted and what the findings were should all be clear to your reader. The discussion enables you to explore the findings from the review in the context of the study as a whole, and the wider literature that is relevant to them. By so doing, it should provide a platform from which you can draw conclusions and make recommendations. To achieve this, the discussion section of your review should:

- highlight the review's key findings, and their importance;
- clarify how the review question was answered and the study aims addressed;
- place the findings within the context of the wider literature;
- evaluate the strengths and limitations of the review and the effect that these had on the findings;
- identify what your study adds to the existing evidence on the subject in question, what is still unknown or unclear, and what requires further investigation (Murray 2011).

The way that you organize the discussion section of your study will, in part, depend on the question and aims that your literature review addressed, and, as a result, there are no absolute rules on how it should be laid out. However, it is generally useful to begin the discussion by providing the reader with a brief synopsis of what will be included in it, and the order in which this will appear (Lunenburg and Irby 2008; White 2011). This enables you to demonstrate that there is system and logic in your decisions about the section, and means that your reader knows what to expect. This brief synopsis is often followed by a summary of the study as a whole, which serves as a concise reminder to your reader of the purpose of your review, its methodology and key findings (Lunenburg and Irby 2008; White 2011).

9.1 Summarizing the review

The summary section of the discussion should not repeat in detail what has already been covered in other parts of your review. Its purpose is to enable your reader to recall the salient points of the story so far, so that these are fresh in their minds as they read the discussion and can see how the study as a whole fits together. The description of the findings, should, for instance, summarize the most important findings, not restate every detail of every finding (White 2011). The most logical way to present these key findings in the summary is usually to link them to the study question or aims (White 2011). This demonstrates to your reader that your study has proceeded in a systematic manner, as it clearly relates the findings to what you set out to discover. For instance, a literature review whose question was: 'How do young people perceive having a long-term neurological condition to affect their engagement in paid employment?' might have aims such as this:

- To ascertain how young people's long-term conditions affect their aspirations for employment.
- To determine whether young people feel that the physical aspects of their condition affect their employment.
- To explore whether non-physical aspects of a long-term condition affect young people's perceived employment experiences.
- To identify whether young people find that people's perceptions of their long-term condition affect their employment.

In the discussion section of the study, this question and these aims could be restated, accompanied by an explanation that the study was, for example, conducted by evaluating literature:

- reporting on qualitative research;
- published between 2006 and 2016;

- related to people aged 16–25;
- that used data from the United Kingdom;
- using the CASP tool for qualitative research;
- using a narrative approach to synthesize the findings from each of the individual papers.

The key findings could then be briefly stated, for instance that:

Whilst not all young people felt that their long-term condition had affected their aspirations for employment, some felt that it had. The reasons for this included specific physical limitations, fatigue, poor self-esteem, and other people's expectations of them. Many young people described how the physical aspects of their condition affected their employment prospects. Some saw this in a negative light, as limiting their opportunities, whilst others viewed it more positively.

Some, but not all, of the young people described specific social and emotional elements of their condition as influencing their employment opportunities. However, it was more common for young people to describe the physical, social and emotional elements of their condition as being linked, not separate entities. The unpredictable nature of their condition was also identified as a common theme throughout all the studies, and as a challenge to young people's initial and ongoing employment.

The effect of other people's attitudes was similarly a common theme across studies, with negative attitudes being seen as rather common. However, whether this was a positive driver to achieve or a detractor from achievement varied. Employers were generally viewed as having positive attitudes towards young people with long-term neurological conditions, although co-workers were not always similarly minded.

This type of brief summary avoids restating the review's methodology and findings in excessive detail, but provides an adequate reminder of its key issues, and enables the reader to proceed through the discussion with these fresh in their mind.

Pitfall to avoid

Avoid restating the full findings of your review in the summary section of your discussion.

9.2 Structuring the main discussion

Having introduced the discussion and briefly summarized the review as a whole, you need to decide how to structure the main part of your discussion. This tends to work best if it mirrors the way in which the results section was laid out, or is structured around the study questions or aims so as to be clearly focused on these (Lunenburg and Irby 2008; White 2011). Depending on how your findings section was presented, you may be able to combine these two approaches. In other cases, you will need to decide which option will work best for your review.

If you decide to structure your discussion around your review question or aims, presenting these in the same order as that in which they were originally presented makes sense, and gives the document as a whole a consistent and logical flow (Lunenburg and Irby 2008). Your discussion will again include a commentary on the findings related to each question or aim. However, they should now be presented in more depth than in the overview, but more concisely than was seen in the results section (Lunenburg and Irby 2008; White 2011). The precise detail of the findings, such as the number of participants in each of the studies, or the statistical tests used in each paper, does not need to be restated. Rather, an overall statement should be made reminding the reader of the key issue that was identified, followed by a discussion of that particular point (Lunenburg and Irby 2008; White 2011).

The discussion section of a literature review concerning the perceived effect of having a long-term neurological condition on young people's employment might begin by exploring the effect that the young person's long-term condition had on their employment aspirations. This could commence with a statement to the effect that the review of the literature showed consistent evidence that a young person's long-term condition affected their career aspirations. This could be followed by a discussion of this finding in the context of other relevant literature in the area, including evidence that fell outside the inclusion criteria, such as case reports, expert opinion or literature from outside the UK. After discussing this general point, particular ways in which young people's aspirations were affected could be highlighted, with each one discussed in detail. The findings from the review, clustered around each of the study questions or aims, thus often form the backbone of the discussion chapter, but they are interrogated, and placed in the context of the wider literature.

Alternatively, if you have presented your findings according to the codes, themes or categories developed in the synthesis process, you may decide to follow this layout to structure your discussion. However, because the intention of the discussion is to focus on what the review has added to the existing body of evidence, it may not be appropriate to include all the codes, themes or categories in the discussion. This decision will depend on what the most important messages from the review are. For example, if there is a category dealing with the methodological issues in the studies included in the review, it may (or may not) be useful to devote a section of the discussion to this. If the section on methodological issues in the study findings merely described and commented on the range of approaches used, and their relative strengths and limitations, it may not be necessary to devote an entire section of the discussion to this. Alternatively, if the review only included qualitative research, but interrogating the study's findings in the context of the wider literature suggests that incorporating quantitative enquiry could have been beneficial, this would probably merit a section in the discussion. Discussing this might, in turn, enable a recommendation to be made for a review that incorporates quantitative evidence to be undertaken. Equally, the discussion of the review's findings might suggest that whilst quantitative perspectives would be a useful addition to the existing evidence base, there is currently a lack of quantitative evidence in this area. This would subsequently enable a recommendation to be made that quantitative research be undertaken in the field of enquiry.

The way in which you structure your discussion should, then, ensure that it clearly relates to the review question, aims and findings, and forms a logical continuation of the previous elements of the study. It should also draw out the contribution that the literature review makes to the existing knowledge base. As a part of this, it should demonstrate how your review fits into, but also augments, the existing relevant literature.

Pitfall to avoid

Avoid making the structure of your discussion so different from other sections of the review that your reader cannot see a logical flow to the document as a whole.

9.3 Comparing the findings from your review to other literature in the field

The discussion section of your literature review must move beyond presenting your findings alongside other information related to the subject to providing an integrated and critically analytical discussion of these (White 2011). A part of achieving this is to evaluate ways in which your study findings corroborate, build on, or differ from, other evidence in the field (Lunenburg and Irby 2008; White 2011).

In your review of the literature, you will have synthesized the findings from the papers included in your study, and determined the overall evidence on the subject in question derived from this process. However, whilst you will have synthesized the evidence from all the papers that met the inclusion criteria for your review, you will not have used all the literature related to this subject area. If you compare the papers on which you carried out the detailed analysis with the background and rationale sections of your review, there will be numerous pieces of evidence in the latter that you will not have included in your synthesis. That will be because some of this was background contextual detail, but other work, whilst being broadly relevant to your study, would not have met your inclusion and exclusion criteria. These latter papers may, nonetheless, be useful to revisit as you discuss your findings and explore how they do, or do not, fit other evidence in the field, and why this may be (Lunenburg and Irby 2008).

The discussion section of the review exploring the experiences of employment of young people with long-term neurological conditions could, for instance, state that the review demonstrated that young people almost universally identified having a long-term condition as affecting their employment aspirations. It might then comment that this is consistent with reports (that were not included in the review) which suggest that young people with long-term conditions may require specific input to enable them to develop and achieve their career aspirations. The discussion could also explore whether evidence from any quantitative research (that was excluded from the review) shows similar findings. This would provide an opportunity for commentary on why any differences in the evidence from different types of research might exist, or how they support and develop one another. Such an approach continues to give primacy of place to the findings from the review, but includes the wider literature in the discussion, and explores key similarities, differences and the reasons for, and importance of, these.

It may also be that literature that is not directly related to your review question is relevant to include in your discussion. For example, a review of the literature might indicate that teachers' perceived attitudes towards young people with long-term neurological conditions were highly influential in the development of their career aspirations. This could then be discussed in light of the more general literature concerning the effect of teachers' perceived attitudes on young people's aspirations. This discussion could include whether the review's findings were similar to those regarding the effect of teachers' perceived attitudes in general, and possible explanations for any differences found. Equally, if you chose to only use literature from the United Kingdom in your review, it might be very useful to include in your discussion how your findings compare to the evidence from studies carried out in other countries. As well as describing the similarities and differences, your discussion should explore why these might exist, and what the implications are for future investigation and practice.

If your findings support other literature, you should highlight this and explain how this strengthens the evidence arising from your work (Lunenburg and Irby 2008). In some cases your review may show findings that are consistent with other work, but also provide more depth of insight into the issues in question. In this situation, you can discuss this, so as to highlight what your study adds to the existing evidence. In other instances, your findings may be at odds with other evidence, in which case you should highlight these differences, and critically discuss why they might exist (Lunenburg and Irby 2008). You can, where appropriate, also use the discussion of the findings to enter into a debate concerning why particular evidence might be missing: for example, why particular types of study, despite their potential value, may not have been carried out.

Pitfall to avoid

Whilst you should include in your discussion how the findings from your review fit within the wider literature, this does not mean that you have to find a way to make your study findings agree with the existing evidence.

9.4 The strengths and limitations of the review

A part of critically discussing the findings from a review is to explore its strengths and limitations, and their probable effects on the findings. Most studies have some limitations. These are not necessarily things that nullify the review's value, or that could have been avoided. They are simply things that in some way limit the scope or extent of the findings. For example, a literature review might use all the available qualitative evidence concerning the career opportunities of young people with long-term neurological conditions. However, there might have been no studies in the review that included young people whose neurological condition severely affected their communication. The review might, in this case, achieve a rigorous and systematic analysis of the existing evidence and draw very sound conclusions. A limitation of the findings would nonetheless be that the evidence from which they were drawn did not include a particular group of the young people with long-term neurological conditions who might have specific employment issues that merit exploration.

To produce a high-quality discussion, it is often ideal if the discussion of the strengths and limitations of your review, and your review's place in the wider literature, can be integrated. In this instance, it would be useful to include in the discussion of this limitation anything that is known from other literature about the effects of having a significant issue with verbal communication, and particularly any information on how this affects young people or people's employment. This would enable the discussion to integrate the findings from the review, their limitations and the wider literature. It would also mean that a conclusion and recommendation regarding the need for research in this area could be made. This appraisal of your own study therefore enables you to clarify precisely what your claims are, and the strength of the conclusions that you can draw, as well as identifying any gaps in the existing evidence.

Other limitations in your study may relate to methodological issues outside your control, such as funding or the number of reviewers available. Again, the effect of these on the study findings, in terms of quality but also the claims that can be made, should be clear. For example, if you were unable to secure resources that would allow translation of papers written in languages that you do not speak, any limitation that this imposed on your study should be discussed. It might be that this posed a significant limitation as three or four potentially relevant articles had to be omitted from the study. Equally, though, your search of the literature may have shown that there were in fact no papers available in other languages. In this latter case, the limitation of excluding non-English language papers would be negligible.

> **Pitfall to avoid**
>
> Avoid trying to gloss over any limitations to your review.
> Acknowledging and discussing these makes your study transparent, analytical and its claims clear.

9.5 Focus on your claims

The discussion section of your study should be limited to the remit of your review. Whilst it should include information other than your data, everything in it should be related to the question and aims that you sought to address, and the findings related to these (White 2011). Additional interesting asides, and ideas not directly relevant to the study question or aims, should not be included. These will obscure the message you are trying to deliver, and leave your study open to the criticism that it is not rigorous and systematic as the discussion encompasses ideas that are not relevant to the question or aims.

Whilst you should exclude any issues that were not a part of your findings from the discussion, if any aspects of your question were not fully answered, or if your aims were incompletely addressed, this should be acknowledged and explored. If, despite including all the research on the subject in question, there was no evidence concerning how the views of other people affected the employment of young people with long-term neurological conditions, this should be clarified in the discussion. In such a situation, explaining that the literature did not include any evidence pertaining to this issue, and thus one study aim could not be fully addressed, would also enable you to recommend that research in this area is needed.

The discussion of the findings from your review should, then, be focused on the study question and aims, and directly related to your findings.

> **Pitfall to avoid**
>
> Avoid introducing new topics areas, or issues not directly related to the study question, aims or findings in the discussion chapter.

Summary

By the end of the discussion chapter your reader should not only know the answer to the review's question and how the aims were met, but also how the findings from the review relate to the wider relevant literature. Your discussion should clarify what you claim that your study adds to the existing evidence, but also the extent and limits of these claims. The claims made should be commensurate with the strength and extent of your findings, neither under nor overstated, and the basis of these claims should be explicit.

The discussion section of your review should be focused around your study question, aims and findings, but needs to go beyond these. The findings should be explored, debated and evaluated in the light of other literature, and the study's strengths and limitations. However, throughout the process, your findings should be the driving force, and it should be clear to your reader what assertions in your discussion are drawn from your findings and what emanates from the wider literature.

Chapter 10

Drawing conclusions and making recommendations

Key points:

- The conclusions drawn and recommendations made from a study that uses literature review methodology should clarify what is now known as a result of the review, and what should be done because of this knowledge.
- The conclusions drawn from the review of the literature should be related to the study question and aims, derived from the findings, and clearly stated.
- The recommendations made should also be grounded in the study findings and arise from the conclusions.

Having completed the findings and discussion sections of your literature review, you are now in a position to state the conclusions that you have drawn, and share the recommendations that arise from these. These conclusions and recommendations should bring your review to a close by providing a clear statement of what is known because the review was conducted, and what should be done because of this (White 2011). The conclusions section is positioned before the recommendations because the recommendations should be made on the basis of what has been concluded.

10.1 The purpose of drawing conclusions

The purpose of the conclusions section of your literature review is exactly what the title suggests: it should draw conclusions from what the review has found. As such, its intention is to demonstrate how the findings have enabled you to answer the study question and address the aims of the review (Lunenburg and Irby 2008). If your literature review has been systematic, with the study question, aims, methods, findings and discussion directly relating to one another, drawing the conclusions should be the next logical step.

The review's question, aims and findings should be the cornerstone of what is concluded, and the conclusions made must be based on evidence that has already been presented in the findings and discussion (White 2011). Writing good quality conclusions therefore requires you to distinguish what the data from your review showed from what this may have made you ponder about. For example, you might have conducted a review that sought to answer the question:

How well do parents who are resident with their child for a planned short stay on a children's ward feel their needs are catered for?

Your aims might, in this case, have been:
- to identify parents' views on how well their physical needs are catered for;
- to understand parents' perceptions of how well their emotional needs are met;
- to determine how well parents feel that their information needs are addressed.

Your findings might have led you to wonder whether there is a gap in pre-registration nurse education regarding catering for resident parents' needs. However, if your data did not actually provide any evidence that education was a factor in how nurses interacted with parents and met their needs, you cannot conclude this. Your review might have made you wonder about it, but you cannot conclude that it is so unless your study demonstrated it to be the case.

Pitfall to avoid

Do not include any points in your conclusions that are not directly related to your findings.

Although the conclusions that you make must be derived from the review's findings and aims, they should not simply reiterate what the findings are, but should explain what they have led you to decide (Lunenburg and Irby 2008). If one of your study aims was to explore parents' perceptions of how well their physical needs were catered for whilst they were staying with their child in hospital, addressing this aim would probably include considering their experiences of accessing meals and refreshments. In your conclusions, rather than reiterating the findings by saying something like:

> All of the papers reviewed indicated that parents found it difficult to take regular meal breaks whilst their child was in hospital. The quantitative studies used Likert-type scales in which median scores related to satisfaction with mealtime provision demonstrated that all parents were either dissatisfied or very dissatisfied. The qualitative studies also showed that parents were not satisfied with their access to meals and refreshments, with every paper providing in-depth quotes that demonstrated that parents' needs were not met in this respect.

Your conclusion should identify what you have decided because of these findings. For instance, you might conclude that:

> Parents being able to take regular breaks for food and refreshments whilst their child was in hospital was highlighted as fraught with difficulties in every study included in this review. Whilst the quality of the studies and their methodological approaches varied, the universality of this finding makes it possible to conclude that gaining adequate access to meals and refreshments is problematic for parents who are resident with their children during planned short-term hospitalization.

Your conclusive statements should also be commensurate with the strength of the evidence from your review (White 2011; Lunenburg and Irby 2008). They should not be overly tentative, nor claim more than the findings from the review merit. If you found something, then claim it, and make it clear to your reader that this was the case. If all the studies that you evaluated demonstrated that parents experience significant difficulty in accessing meals and refreshments during their child's hospital stay, you can confidently conclude that the review has shown this to be the case. However, if the composite evidence was that some parents, especially younger parents, found it difficult to leave their child in order to get meals, but that others did not find this to be a problem, then your claim should be more moderate. It might perhaps be something to the effect that the review concludes that parents, and especially younger parents, can experience difficulties in gaining access to meals. You should also be clear about the population or circumstances to which your conclusions apply (White 2011; Lunenburg and Irby 2008). If your review only included parents whose children were hospitalized short term, for a planned admission, this is the population to whom you can conclude that your findings apply.

Pitfall to avoid

Avoid being overly tentative or grandiose with your conclusions: claim exactly what your findings showed.

10.2 Developing good quality conclusions

Developing clear and relevant conclusions can be harder than it seems. When you plan your review it is therefore worth ensuring that you have set aside enough time to carefully consider and write these.

Your conclusions should be focused on the review's question and aims, so if you find yourself writing a conclusion about something that is not related to either of these, you should probably consider very carefully whether it should be there. There may of course be situations where you have found something important that was not one of the aims of your review, and, because of its significance, feel that it should be afforded the prominence that a conclusion has. New knowledge should not be resisted just because you did not intend to find it. However, the vast majority of your conclusions should be related to a study question or aim, and should always be derived from the findings. The presence of any conclusions that fall outside the study aims should be justified, and their inclusion should not be at the expense of addressing the aims of the review.

A second point to check when writing your conclusions is that each one is based on judgements that can reasonably be made because of the findings from the review (White 2011). To achieve this, it can be helpful to ask yourself, as you draw each conclusion: 'Where in the findings was this shown?'. If the answer is that you have not shown it in the findings, it should probably not feature in the conclusions.

The golden rule is, then, that your conclusions should be based on what your review showed. This includes any instances where your study demonstrated that there was a lack of evidence on a particular matter. Your review may, for instance, have found that there is very little evidence concerning how well parents' emotional needs are addressed whilst they are resident with their hospitalized child. In this case, one of your conclusions would be that at present there is limited evidence concerning how well parents' emotional needs are met.

As this chapter will go on to discuss, this type of conclusion would lend itself to a recommendation that, because of the current lack of evidence, there is a need for primary research to be conducted in the area in question.

There may also be situations where the evidence on a subject is inconclusive or contradictory. It can be tempting to try to explain away this type of uncertainty, and to create a conclusion that provides a clear yes or no answer. However, if a mixed or uncertain picture is what the review of the literature showed, that is what you must conclude, because your task is to draw conclusions that are faithfully based on what was found. For example, if the evidence from the papers that you reviewed is that mothers were more likely to have their mealtime needs met than fathers, then this is your conclusion. However, if there were quite marked differences in how well parents perceived their mealtime needs to be met, but no particular characteristics in the participants involved, nature or quality of the studies that would account for this, your conclusion should reflect this uncertainty. You could conclude that some parents' needs for meal and refreshment breaks are met well, whilst others are not, but that the reasons for these differences are not clear, and cannot be accounted for by the characteristics of the study populations, research design or quality. A conclusion that might be drawn in such a situation could be:

> Parents may experience difficulty in accessing adequate meal and refreshment breaks whilst resident with their hospitalized child. The factors that predispose to this merit further investigation, but as there is currently no conclusive evidence regarding these, it should be considered a risk for all parents.

Pitfall to avoid

There is a need for clarity in your conclusions, but not for portrayal of a certainty that does not exist.

In addition to the key criteria of addressing the study question and aims, and being directly informed by the study findings, the conclusions should be clear, concise and specific. Each should be presented in a manner that provides a reasoned, evidence-based, summary judgement on the point in question (White 2011). The depth of discussion that you enter into for each point will depend on the purpose of your review and the wordage available to you. If your review is being conducted to fulfil the requirements of an academic dissertation, you will need to go well beyond presenting your conclusions as a series of bullet points. Instead, it will be necessary for you to demonstrate a clear, and analytical, reason for drawing the conclusions that you have.

Your conclusions should be clearly articulated and well reasoned, but they do not need to be extensive in number. A small number of conclusions that relate directly to your review question and aims, are derived from your findings, and consistent with the strength and scope of your evidence, is preferable to an extensive list of ideas, many of which are not related to the focus of your review. If your conclusions are derived from your findings and clearly stated, they form a good basis from which to make your recommendations.

> **Pitfall to avoid**
>
> It is the quality, rather than quantity, of your conclusions that really matters.

10.3 Determining the recommendations from the review

Having presented your conclusions, the final element of your review is to use these to make recommendations that state what actions should be taken because of them. These actions can be things that you recommend should be undertaken by government, policymakers, local service providers or individual staff, and may concern research, education, policy or practice. Regardless of the target group for action, they, like the conclusions, should have a specific focus and scope. For example, the recommendations from a review whose aim was to explore the experiences of parents whose children were electively hospitalized short term should be focused on that group. Even if you think that the recommendations you are making could usefully be applied more widely, if that was the population included in your review, it is as far as your recommendations can go. The exception is if you are recommending further research or reviews that include a wider population.

Because recommendations concern things that should be done, they should be achievable (Lunenburg and Irby 2008). For example, the evidence from your review might be that parents feel unable to take meal breaks because the nurses appear to be too busy to sit with their child whilst they are away. This might have led you to conclude that the perceived busyness of nursing staff is a contributor to parents feeling unable to access adequate meals or refreshments. A recommendation that nurses should make themselves available to sit with children so as to provide parents with breaks might, in this case, seem desirable. However, it might also be unachievable. A more achievable recommendation might be that alternative options for providing refreshments for parents be considered, such as vending machines or facilities for parents to prepare basic meals and make beverages being available on wards.

Pitfall to avoid

Avoid recommending actions that it would be impossible to achieve.

Because many studies raise additional questions as well as providing answers, there are almost always recommendations for further research at the end of a study (Lunenburg and Irby 2008). However, these recommendations should, like the other recommendations made, be specific, and based on the conclusions that have been drawn. For instance, your conclusions might include that there is a lack of clarity over the factors that predispose parents whose children are in hospital short term, for a planned admission, having poor access to meals. A recommendation might in this case be that more research should be conducted into the mealtime needs of parents whose children are in hospital short term for a planned admission. It should not indicate that this research is needed for a wider population, as your review has not shown this to be the case. Like the conclusions, the recommendations from your literature review should be firmly grounded in the findings from your study, and based on that evidence, not your opinion or experience (Lunenburg and Irby 2008).

The recommendations for further study may include questions that have arisen from the limitations in your review (Lunenburg and Irby 2008). If you noted, on reflection, that including additional databases or keywords would have enhanced the review, you might recommend that the review be repeated using these databases or keywords. Equally, if you had no funding for translation services, but know that this resulted in several papers being omitted from your review, you might recommend that the review be repeated with the inclusion of languages other than English.

The recommendations should, therefore, be succinct, focused, achievable statements that clarify what should be done because of the conclusions that have been drawn in the study.

Summary

The mainstay of a good literature review is that it is rigorous and systematic. The conclusions and recommendations sections of a study that uses literature review methodology are no exception to this rule. They should be the logical end point of the research question, aims, methodology, methods, findings and discussion of the findings. Each conclusion should be clearly recognizable as the logical outcome of a study finding, and linked to a study question or aim. Similarly, each recommendation should be an action that is associated with one of the conclusions drawn from the literature review. Each recommendation should also be achievable, and commensurate with the strength of the findings and conclusion on which it is based.

The conclusions and recommendations are a very important part of your study, being the summary statements of all your work, drawing it to a close, but also opening up the findings from the study so that the reader sees what they mean and what can be done with them (Lunenburg and Irby 2008). They should provide your reader with a clear vision of what your study found, what this means, and what should be done because of it. However, whilst the conclusions and recommendations should show the importance of your literature review, they should not make any claims beyond what your study showed.

Key points:

- Disseminating the findings from studies that use literature review methodology enables others to understand what the current best evidence on a subject is.
- Publishing the findings from a literature review in a journal or presenting them at a conference are two options for sharing the knowledge that you have gained as a result of conducting your study.
- Using online social media is becoming an increasingly important way of sharing the findings from studies.

Having carried out your literature review, you will almost certainly have information that it would be useful for others to know about. One of the reasons why you undertook a review of the literature is likely to have been that the composite best evidence on the subject in question required clarification. The chances are, therefore, that someone else will also be interested to know what the evidence from across sources is, and if you now know this, it makes sense to share that information.

If the findings from your review of the literature were that the current evidence on a particular subject is inconclusive, you may feel that sharing this information is of no real benefit. However, the opposite is true. If you have found that the existing evidence on a subject is not clear-cut, making this information available will establish what is and is not known, overall, about the subject, and the quality of that evidence. Knowing that there is a lack of strong evidence concerning a particular subject will enable practitioners to make decisions with clients based on a realistic evaluation of what is and is not known, and the certainty with which it is known. It will also highlight, for both practitioners and researchers, areas where further research might be useful.

> **Pitfall to avoid**
>
> The findings from a review that has shown there to be contradictory or poor quality evidence on a subject merit sharing just as much as those from a review that has demonstrated consistency and clarity in the existing evidence. Knowing what evidence does, but also does not, exist in a particular field of practice is likely to be very useful.

Usually, therefore, if you have carried out a study that used literature review methodology, however small the scale of your review, it will be worth sharing your findings. There are a number of approaches to getting information about your work into the public domain, three of which are written publications, conference presentations and using online social media.

11.1 Publication

One option for sharing the findings from your literature review is to write a paper for a relevant journal. The first step in this process is to decide what key message you want to share, and the audience that you want to communicate your message to. Although your literature review will have been very focused, you may still need to make a decision as to whether there is a particular aspect of it that is the priority for you to disseminate information about. For example, if you had carried out a literature review related to the quality of mealtime provision for older people on acute medical wards, you might have findings related to the quality of food offered, and the way in which people were enabled to partake in meals. Both of these aspects of your findings would be important. However, you might decide that you wanted to focus on sharing information about the way in which people are enabled to partake in the experience of having a meal.

As well as determining the precise remit of your article, you will need to decide on your target audience: for instance, whether this will be frontline practitioners, academics, or both (Glasper and Peate 2013). Within these broad categories, you may want to focus even more specifically on one particular group, for example those in a specific area of practice, or those from one profession (Happell 2008). Making these decisions will enable you to identify journals that are appropriate for your target audience. If your review concerned the quality of mealtime provision for older people on acute medical wards you might primarily want to share the evidence concerning what nurses can do to enhance people's mealtime experiences. Although your findings relate to older people on acute medical wards, the messages that you have to share might be sufficiently applicable to nurses in other areas of practice for you to choose to write for a general nursing journal. Equally, your decision could be that as your review concerned older people you would prefer to write for a journal that focuses on this client group. Making these decisions means that you can identify the publication that you are interested in contributing to, and tailor your writing to that journal's requirements, rather than preparing your work in a style that you will subsequently have to alter.

Having identified journals that might be suitable for you to write for, the next step is to access their information for authors. This will provide you with information concerning the journal's target audience, what types of article are usually published, how the manuscript should be presented, and how many words an article should be (Glasper and Peate 2013; Bingham 2014). Looking at these, and a recent edition of the journal, will help you to assess the style, tone and approach used, and to decide whether this matches what you want to present.

If you are unsure about whether a report from a study that used literature review methodology is something that a particular journal will accept, you can contact the editor to check this. If you are in any doubt about whether what you aim to present will meet the journal's remit, it is well worth making such an enquiry. This saves you the time and effort of preparing a manuscript that complies with the requirements of a particular journal, only to have your paper rejected because it is not something that the journal would publish, regardless of its quality.

Pitfall to avoid

Avoid writing a complete manuscript before checking the word count, style and subject material that the journal of your choice will accept.

When you write for publication, you will need to plan exactly what will be included in your article, and the key messages that you want to deliver. Usually, the layout for a report on a study that used literature review methodology will follow the same format that the review itself did:

• The background and rationale for the review
• The review question

- The aims and objectives of the review
- The methods of carrying out the search
- The methods used to appraise the literature
- The way in which the synthesis of the appraised literature was performed
- The findings from the review
- A discussion of the review's findings
- The conclusions
- The recommendations.

Looking at the usual layout of articles in the journal that you hope to contribute to and checking the guidelines for authors will, however, enable you to gauge how reports should be structured for that specific journal (Glasper and Peate 2013).

Having planned what you will write, the mechanism of preparing the manuscript itself will closely resemble the process that you have gone through to write your review of the literature. It is usually best to write a plan or outline, then a draft manuscript, followed by reviewing and editing the draft until you are satisfied that the content is focused, covers your key points, and is presented in a logical order (Bingham 2014). The time that it may take to rewrite your study for the purpose of publication should not be underestimated. If you have completed your initial literature review as the dissertation element of a programme of academic study, you will have significantly fewer words at your disposal when writing for publication. Deciding which of the elements of the review can be omitted, without losing your key messages or detracting from the sense of the rigour of your study, can be a time-consuming process.

Whilst a journal article cannot contain a detailed account of everything that you did, it should provide a clear enough description of the steps you took for the reader to be convinced that your review was systematic and rigorous. Therefore, whilst being concise, your article also needs to be logical, and take the reader step-by-step through the process and outcomes of your study. There may be aspects of your methodology that can be concisely summarized using tables or figures, such as a list of the databases searched and a flow diagram of the number of papers identified. Such tables or figures can be a useful means of presenting key information, but they need to be signposted from your main text, so that your reader understands their place in your report.

Before you submit your manuscript to a journal, it is worth asking a trusted colleague, peer or friend, who will be supportively but constructively critical, to read it. This can help you to gauge whether someone who has not been immersed in the study, as you will have been, can follow your decision trail and argument (Glasper and Peate 2013; Bingham 2014).

Once you have submitted your manuscript to the journal of your choice it will be reviewed. Many journals use a process of peer review, meaning that at least one (and usually two or three) experts assess the quality of the manuscript. Some journals use a double blind peer review process, in which the writer's and reviewers' identities are not disclosed to each other. Others use open peer review, where the reviewers' and writer's identities are available to one another. Being peer reviewed generally means that a journal is more highly regarded than if it were not, as it provides some assurance that the articles in it are deemed to be of good quality.

The journal's reviewers will decide whether your manuscript should be accepted as it is, that revisions should be made to it, or whether it lacks the essential quality requirements for publication. In addition, reviewers may sometimes decide that whilst a paper is of good quality it is not suitable for the particular journal in question, and recommend that it be submitted elsewhere. It is very common to be asked to make revisions to a manuscript, and this should be regarded as the next stage of writing rather than a failure (Bingham 2014). If you are asked to make revisions, it indicates that the reviewers consider your work to be of sufficient quality and importance to merit publication, but that it requires some work to ensure that it gives a clear message and showcases your work to its best advantage.

Pitfall to avoid

If you are asked to make revisions to your manuscript, do not regard this as a failure. It means that your work is considered likely to make a valuable contribution, but requires a little more input in order to do itself justice.

Whilst writing a journal article is a very good way of disseminating the findings from a literature review, it is not the only option available to you. You may, instead, decide to present your work at a conference.

11.2 Conference presentations

Presenting at a conference is a useful way of sharing the findings from your literature review. If you decide that this is an option that you wish to explore, you will, in the same way as you would with a written publication, need to make a decision about what the key messages that you want to deliver are, and the audience to whom you would like to present your work.

If you apply to present your literature review at a conference, you will usually be given the choice of a poster or concurrent oral presentation as your preferred medium. Both options are useful opportunities to share your work, and the choice you make will probably depend on the material you want to present and how you would prefer to deliver your message. In both cases, when you submit your application (usually in the form of an abstract) you should be clear about what your key messages will be, and how these fit the conference's remit. As with planning a paper for publication in a journal, you may decide that in order to present in adequate depth, and within the time or space allowed, you will focus on a particular aspect of your literature review. As well as being what the reviewers use to make a decision about your application, the abstract that you submit will be what the conference delegates read when they decide whether or not to attend your session or visit your poster. The information contained in it therefore needs to be engaging, match the remit of the conference, and precisely reflect the key messages that you will ultimately present (Happell 2009). For instance, if you applied to present the findings from a review concerning the quality of mealtime provision for older people on acute medical wards at a conference related to humanizing care, your abstract would need to demonstrate that the concept of humanization would be a central part of your presentation. You would also need to ensure that this was reflected in what you subsequently prepared and presented.

11.2.1 Oral presentations

If you are invited to deliver an oral presentation at a conference, you should check what format this is expected to take, how long you have for your presentation, whether this includes time for questions, and what equipment will be available to you. The letter indicating that your abstract has been accepted will usually include these details, and, having ascertained this information, you then need to plan your presentation.

A concurrent oral presentation session is usually relatively short, so you will need to strike the balance between demonstrating the rigour of your study, capturing your audience's interest, and avoiding trying to cram in too much information (Happell 2009). To achieve this, you should use a logical structure that leads the listener through your decisions. However, you should also bear in mind that the people who choose to attend your session are likely to do so because they have some knowledge about or interest in the subject. Therefore, whilst you need to provide a short background to the study, unless the remit of your presentation is the methodological approach used, the focus should be on the new knowledge that your study has brought to the field: your findings, conclusions and recommendations (Happell 2009). These should also be related to the conference's remit. If, for example, the conference theme is humanization of care, how the findings, conclusions and recommendations that you focus on link to the humanization agenda need to be very clear.

Pitfall to avoid

Avoid trying to pack everything from your review into a short presentation slot. Decide what your priority is, and make this the focus of your presentation.

As well as the content of your presentation, its visual impact is important. Any slides that you use need to be legible, and not over-crowded (Happell 2009). In terms of how you present, there is no one right way to speak at a conference: this depends on what you are comfortable with, your experience and confidence. If you are unused to presenting in public it is usually useful to write a full paper detailing exactly what you will say in your presentation. Even if you do not intend to read from this, it is useful to have as an emergency backup in case, on the day, you need a prompt (Happell 2009). It can also be useful to think about what questions people may ask, and have spare notes or slides that deal with anticipated queries. For instance, you may have decided that in order to focus on your findings you will only give a brief overview of the details of the methodology of your review. In this situation, you could ensure that you have to hand a reminder of which databases you searched, and the keywords and synonyms that you used, in case someone asks about these. However familiar you are with your study it is always possible that when you are asked a question your mind will go blank, and having additional slides or notes can be a useful guard against this.

Pitfall to avoid

If you are giving an oral presentation at a conference, make sure that you have notes to read from as a backup.

Asking someone who will give supportive but critical feedback to listen to you rehearsing your presentation can be very helpful (Happell

2009). Even if they know nothing about your subject you will be able to obtain feedback on whether your flow of ideas is logical, can be followed, makes sense to someone who has not been involved with your work, and if the pace of your speech is right. It also means that you can realistically gauge whether what you plan to present matches the time that you have been allocated.

11.2.2 Poster presentations

If you are invited to present a poster at a conference, you will be provided with guidelines on the format and size that posters should conform to, and the timings of the poster sessions (Christenbery and Latham 2013). Like other presentation options, posters need to be carefully planned, including the key messages you aim to deliver in a relatively small physical space (Hess *et al.* 2009).

Although the timing of poster viewings is more flexible than the time allocated to an oral presentation, most conference delegates will only spend a short time at each poster, so your aim should be to attract them to your work with a compelling style and message (Christenbery and Latham 2013). If your poster is crowded, or uses a lot of small writing so as to fit in as much information as possible, people may not find it attractive to look at, and thus may not feel encouraged to view it. In contrast, if your poster looks engaging, and has a title that attracts interest, you will be able to discuss additional details about your work with the people who are drawn to it. Ideally, your aim should be to have a mix of interesting and relevant illustrations and related but concisely written statements that make people want to learn more about your work (Christenbery and Latham 2013). For example, trying to list all the keywords, synonyms, Boolean operators, etc. that you used in your review would usually take up too much space on a poster and make it cluttered. Anyone who is interested in your review can ask you about these. For the purpose of a poster, the study question, and that it used literature review methodology, is likely to be sufficient background detail. The focus should be on what you found, and what your conclusions are. As with an oral presentation, it is useful to have a report on your review to hand to provide prompts from which you can discuss particular points with people who express an interest in your work.

Pitfall to avoid

Avoid trying to cram too much information onto a poster.

Finally, it is worth planning ahead to the production stage of your poster at an early point. This includes deciding how you will have the poster produced, and checking the timing and cost of this, so as to ensure that you have the requisite materials with the necessary party in plenty of time.

Whilst publishing in journals and presenting at conferences have traditionally been the mainstays of disseminating the findings from studies, it is becoming increasingly common to also use electronic social media to share this type of information.

11.3 Electronic social media

Using electronic social media is becoming a valuable way of disseminating new knowledge. Like all methods of disseminating information, using this approach to sharing the findings from your literature review has strengths and limitations. Disseminating information electronically is a very prompt way of sharing the outcomes of studies with a potentially very wide audience (McGeehan *et al.* 2009; Cann 2011; Rowlands *et al.* 2011). However, it should also be approached with a degree of caution, and requires knowledge of whom you are sharing with, and how secure the information that you share is (Cann 2011). Social media (such as Twitter, Facebook or blogging) enable you to share headline news about your findings, conclusions and recommendations. However, these approaches do not allow the in-depth description and analysis that, for example, writing a journal article does. They do, nonetheless, allow those seeking and sharing information to discuss it, ask questions, and seek clarifications in a way that some other approaches do not (Cann 2011). They can also be a useful means of highlighting what you have published, presented, or aim to present, so that people who are interested know where they can find out more.

As with all other methods of sharing information, your decision about whether or not to include electronic social media in your dissemination plan depends on what information you want to share, the audience you want to share it with, and what you feel will be the best way of achieving this.

Summary

Having completed your review of the literature, it is usually very useful if you can disseminate the findings from your study. Doing this means that other people have the chance to see an overview of what the current best evidence on a subject is, rather than having to repeat the process of reviewing the literature that you have already undertaken. The two traditional ways of sharing findings from studies have been publication and conference presentations. However, using online social media is becoming an increasingly important way of sharing new knowledge. Your decision concerning how you will disseminate the findings from your literature review should be guided by what would best suit the message you want to deliver, and how confident you feel about using each option. Having said that, disseminating the findings from your review can also be an opportunity to move slightly outside your comfort zone, in terms of trying a new approach.

Carrying out a study that uses literature review methodology is a very valuable way of collating the existing knowledge in a field of practice, as it enables what is, and is not, known about a subject to be clarified. However, for a literature review to make a useful and meaningful contribution to the evidence base it must be conducted systematically, rigorously and without bias (Cronin *et al.* 2008; Aveyard 2014: 3–4). Whilst exactly how a literature review is conducted will depend on the question that the review seeks to answer, there are particular steps that should be taken in order to assist in the study in achieving these quality standards.

The reason for deciding to undertake the literature review in question should be made clear by the presentation of a focused, unbiased background to and rationale for the study. This should include relevant literature related to the subject in question, but can also incorporate practice-based and personal reasons for undertaking the review. This section of the review should bring the reader to a point at which the study question and aims are the logical next step.

The question that the review seeks to answer should be precise, focused, and clearly related to the background and rationale for the study. This is, arguably, one of the most important parts of the review, as it is the foundation on which the study as a whole rests. The review question is usually followed by the aims of the study. These should detail precisely what the review intends to achieve in order to answer its question. Many studies also include objectives that outline what will be done in order to achieve the aims. The review question, aims and objectives should therefore form a natural, intrinsically linked, sequence: fulfilling the objectives will mean that the aims are met, and addressing the aims will enable the review question to be answered. These three parts of the review being consistent with one another contributes to the review being rigorous and systematic. In addition, if the question, aims and objectives of the review are well defined, and link directly to one another, it will assist in the development of systematic and rigorous methods for the review, because what these need to be designed to achieve will be clear.

The methods used in a study that uses literature review methodology essentially detail the process of searching for, appraising and synthesizing the evidence on the subject in question. These processes should be consistent with the study question, aims and objectives, and conducted rigorously, systematically and without bias. Any frameworks or tools used to assist in conducting the review should be selected because of their quality, and their congruence with the review question, aims, objectives, inclusion and exclusion criteria.

Once the information from across the papers included in the review has been synthesized, the findings from the study should be presented in a manner that indicates how the review question has been answered and the aims met. This presentation of the findings should be followed by a discussion of these, in which the strengths and limitations of the review, their effect on the findings, and how the findings fit the wider context within which the study was conducted should be presented.

Finally, the report from a study that uses literature review methodology should present conclusions that are firmly grounded in the review's findings, and address its question and aims, followed by recommendations that are based on these conclusions.

The stages described above form the key components of a study that uses literature review methodology. However, in order for the study as a whole to be of good quality each step needs to be conducted systematically, rigorously, and in a manner that reduces to a minimum the risk of the apparent findings being due to bias or an error in the process of enquiry. In addition, there needs to be a sense of coherence and continuity of decision-making between the sections.

When a rigorous and systematic review of the literature on a particular subject has been carried out, it will usually be useful for the knowledge generated from it to be shared. This will enable what is and is not known on the subject, and the strength of the existing evidence, to become more widely known and acted upon. It allows direction for current practice, and enables practitioners to work with clients to make informed choices, based on a realistic understanding of the current evidence base. It also enables any gaps in the current knowledge base to be identified, and, by so doing, highlights areas where additional investigation could be useful.

Carrying out a study that uses literature review methodology can, therefore, be a valuable contribution to knowledge. However, the worth of a literature review, like any other form of research, is dependent on its quality.

Troubleshooting guide

The following guide suggests solutions to difficulties that are commonly encountered in the course of conducting a study that uses literature review methodology. Where appropriate, it provides links to chapters where the issue in question is discussed in more detail.

1 I've got too many ideas

This is quite a common problem at the start of any type of research, because every subject has a huge range of possibilities that could be explored.

One way to resolve this problem is to write down all your ideas, and then decide which ones you really want to explore. Consider which of these ideas really appeal to you, and which are interesting, but not compelling. If you have a lot of ideas, it may be useful to list them in order of the level of interest that they hold for you. This could be a professional interest, a personal interest, or what your workplace needs you to do at present.

Whilst an interest in your subject is essential, competing issues often also need to be taken into account. Although you might find something very interesting, your workplace may require you to explore something else as a part of your role. If you cannot do both, you will need to decide which will take priority at this point in time.

Therefore, if you have too many ideas, you may find it useful to narrow your ideas down by creating a shortlist that you can then place in order of interest or priority. The one that is highest on the list is probably the one that you should pursue.

2 I can't decide what my review question is

As Chapters 3 and 5 discuss, to achieve a good quality review it is important to have a very clearly focused question and aims. Therefore, if you cannot decide what the question that you want to address in your review is, you should spend some time on this before moving on to the next stages in your study.

To decide what your question is, first determine your general topic area (as described in the first point of this guide), then consider everything which that broad subject includes. For example, if you are interested in the uptake of the influenza vaccination, you could think about what this topic area encompasses: the uptake amongst specific age groups, the uptake in particular geographical areas, etc. Having decided which aspect or aspects of the topic you want to focus on, the next step is to make this area of interest into a question.

If you decided that you were interested in the uptake of the influenza vaccination in people aged over seventy-five, you might want to focus on what currently acts as a barrier or facilitator to people in this age group accessing the vaccination. Your question might then be:

> What are the barriers and facilitators to people aged over seventy-five receiving the influenza immunization?

You might also want to consider whether you wish to limit this question to a particular geographical area, such as the United Kingdom, in which case, your question might be:

> What are the barriers and facilitators to people aged over seventy-five who live in the United Kingdom receiving the influenza immunization?

3 My topic seems too narrow

Thinking that your topic is too narrow is quite common, but this often turns out not to be a problem at all. As Chapters 4 and 5 identify, it is more common to have to narrow your focus than to expand it.

If you think that your topic is too narrow the best thing to do is to find out whether it is or not. Otherwise, you may expand it, only to have to narrow it again. To do this, develop your search strategy as described in Chapter 6 and carry out an initial search. If you get too few papers, check to see if:

- there are any sources of information, such as additional databases, that you have not included;
- there are any keywords or synonyms that you have omitted;
- you have used Boolean operators appropriately;
- you have inadvertently searched in too narrow a field.

If you feel convinced that your search was comprehensive, but you still have too few papers, then perhaps your topic is indeed too narrow. In this case, you should return to your question and decide what aspect of it could be expanded.

4 My topic seems too broad

This is a very common problem, and many studies begin by having too broad a remit. One way to address this, as Chapter 5 and point two of this guide outline, is to think about what the topic that you have chosen includes. This will provide you with some idea as to whether or not it needs to be broken down so as to become more focused. If it does, once you have identified the key aspects of the topic, you can decide which of these more specific aspects of the subject you really want to explore. You may also need to consider whether this more focused area can itself be broken down into an even narrower question.

5 I get confused between aims and objectives

As Chapter 5 outlines, the aims of a study are what the study intends to achieve, and the objectives are what will be done to enable those aims to be achieved. Meeting the aims will enable the review question to be answered, and fulfilling the objectives will enable the aims to be achieved. Neither should go beyond the scope of your question and both should be achievable.

6 I can't access the full text of all the articles that my search produced

Although many journal articles are available as electronic full text options, either via a university's online library, your employer's library facilities or as online open access articles, some are not. In this situation, your university or employer's library can usually obtain these for you through the interlibrary loans system. Interlibrary loans are often delivered electronically, but retrieving them can take some time, so it is important to plan ahead and order any papers that you may need to access this way in a timely manner. There may also be restrictions on how many interlibrary loans any individual can order, so it is worth checking if such a limit exists, and, if necessary, considering which articles are vital for your review. In many cases you can view the abstracts of papers online even if the full text is not available, which enables you to assess whether any particular article is one that you really need.

7 I haven't found enough articles

If your initial search has not returned enough articles for the purpose of your review, you should review your decisions to see if there are any additional:

- databases;
- keywords;
- synonyms

that you could include in your search. You should also check whether the field that you have chosen to search in is wide enough (for example, you may wish to search in the article's title, keywords and abstract rather than just in the title). Revisiting how you have used Boolean operators, especially the 'not' operator, to ensure that you have not inadvertently excluded relevant studies is also advisable.

If, after reviewing these decisions, you are confident that you have gathered all the available evidence on your chosen subject, but that this is not enough to carry out a study using literature review methodology, you may need to broaden your inclusion and exclusion criteria. For example, you could decide to include more types of literature, more locations or a wider time frame. If you still have very little literature, you may need to revisit your review question and consider how you can make this slightly broader.

8 I have found too many articles

If your search has returned more papers than you will be able to meaningfully sift through, you should revisit your keywords and synonyms to check whether these include any words that, in fact, fall outside the remit of your review. You should also check whether you have made the best use of Boolean operators, and if you have searched in the right fields. If you are confident that your search itself is sufficiently narrow, but you still have an unmanageable volume of literature, you need to consider how you can narrow your focus. First, you could revisit the inclusion and exclusion criteria, and consider further limiting the type of literature, date, language or location of studies that will be incorporated in the review. If, after taking this step, you still have too many results to be manageable, you will probably need to revisit your question and narrow its focus as outlined in point four of this guide.

9 Should this article be included in my review?

If you are not sure whether a particular article that you have retrieved should be included in your review, return to your inclusion and exclusion criteria. If the paper does not meet your inclusion criteria, and/or falls within your exclusion criteria then it should not be included. If it meets your inclusion criteria and does not fall within your exclusion criteria, it should be included.

10 Is this paper good enough to be included in the review?

Generally speaking, all the papers that you retrieve that meet the study's inclusion criteria and do not fall within the exclusion criteria should be included in the review. You will comment on the quality and the strength of the evidence provided in each study in your findings and discussion sections, and these will influence how much weight each study is afforded in the review's findings, conclusions and recommendations. Occasionally, you will find that a particular study is of such poor quality that its evidence does not merit inclusion in your findings. However, the paper itself should still be included in the review and the reason for its evidence being omitted from the findings explained.

The only reason for excluding a paper from the review based on its quality is if one of the study's inclusion criteria is a particular quality indicator and the paper in question does not meet that criterion.

11 I can't decide if this article is research or not

Ideally, an article that reports on research should describe itself as such, by:

- using the term 'research'
  or
- using a term that refers to a particular research paradigm or methodology such as 'qualitative', 'quantitative', 'mixed methods', 'positivist', 'interpretivist', 'grounded theory', 'phenomenology', 'ethnography'

or

- by explaining the study design, e.g. 'randomized controlled trial', 'case control study', 'cohort study'.

However, if such terms are not evident, but you still think the paper may be a research report, you should look at its structure. If it includes subheadings that suggest that a research process was used, such as methodology, methods, findings, it may well be a report on research. However, it may equally be a report on an audit or evaluation. A useful guide as to whether a paper reports on audit, evaluation or research may be to remember that:

- research investigates what should be done;
- audit investigates whether or not what should be done is being done;
- evaluation examines how useful or effective something is, or what standard it achieves (National Health Service Health Research Authority 2009, revised 2013).

12 I can't decide which tool to use to evaluate the papers for my review

As Chapter 7 identifies, any tool that you decide to use needs to be one that will work for your particular review: it should be one that is designed for use with the type of paper you are evaluating, and which you feel you can work with. If your review includes a variety of different study designs, you may decide to use a fairly generic tool, so that you can use the same one for all the papers in your review. Alternatively, you may decide to use a different tool for each type of study or evidence that is included in your review.

It is sensible to only use tools that are established as being of good quality in your review. Using a poor quality tool would mean that the decisions into which the tool guided you might be flawed.

13 Do I need a table for my findings?

You do not absolutely need a table for your findings, because the use of tables is very much dependent upon the question that your study seeks to address, the type of evidence you have included, and, to some extent, your personal presentation preferences. However, it will usually be useful to have a table summarizing the papers included in the review, their key characteristics, findings, strengths and limitations. You will also often find that it is useful to summarize other key issues in your study by using a table or diagram. For example, a flow diagram might be used to demonstrate how you conducted your search: how many papers each database returned; how many duplicate papers were found; how many papers that were retrieved were subsequently found not to meet the review's inclusion criteria; and therefore how you ended up with the papers that you did for your review.

When you consider whether or not you need a table or diagram at any point in your study, ask yourself: would a table or diagram help my reader to understand what I did, or what I am explaining? Remember to signpost your reader to all your tables and diagrams so that they can see how these contribute to your review.

14 My discussion chapter seems like a repeat of my findings chapter

Your discussion chapter or section should, as Chapter 9 outlines, be focused on the findings from the review, but should interpret, develop and explore these in light of the wider literature and the strengths and limitations of your study. If you are unsure whether you have achieved this, you can check whether:

- your statements about the findings as presented in the discussion are more succinct than they were in the findings section of your review;
- you have discussed how each of the findings compares with the wider literature on the subject;
- you have highlighted how the strengths and limitations of your review may have influenced the findings.

Your discussion section or chapter may have similar or identical subheadings to the findings section or chapter, but the content of the discussion section should analyse your findings in the context of the study as a whole, and in light of other literature in the field.

15 My conclusions seem a bit weak

As Chapter 10 discusses, your conclusions should be clear statements of what is now known because of your review. The strength of each of your conclusions should be commensurate with the strength of the evidence in your findings. Regardless of the strength of your evidence though, your conclusions should be clear, decisive and make a claim, even if that claim is that there is currently little evidence about a particular matter.

16 How do I know if my review is biased?

Some steps that you can take to check whether your review is biased include checking the following:

- Have you proved a point that you started out wanting to prove? If so, make sure that your data have led you to this conclusion rather than you leading your data to that conclusion.
- Have you omitted the findings from any of the papers included in the review from the review's findings? If so, is your rationale for this clear?
- Have you given appropriate weight to the findings from each study?
- Is the quality of each paper what has led you to attribute the value that you have to its findings?
- Have you included both sides of the story where the evidence from across sources is mixed?
- Has your discussion critically analysed your findings, and the strengths and limitations of the review?
- Do your conclusions arise directly from your findings and the discussion of these?
- Are your recommendations a natural outcome of your conclusions?

17 How do I know if my review is systematic and rigorous?

Some ways to check whether your review is systematic and rigorous include asking yourself these questions:

- Do the background and rationale for the review lead logically to my review question?
- Do the background and rationale show why literature review methodology was an appropriate approach to use for my study?
- Are my study question, aims and objectives logical continuations of one another?
- Do my keywords reflect the review question?
- Were the synonyms of my keywords systematically developed?
- Were Boolean operators (if used) applied appropriately?
- Did my search include all the relevant databases?
- Are the limits of my search clear and reasoned?
- Did my inclusion and exclusion criteria enable me to include all the literature relevant to my review question and aims, and exclude all irrelevant literature?
- Were the appraisal tools or processes that I used suitable for the type of literature in question?
- Did I use the appraisal tools or processes that I selected consistently across all the papers included in my review?
- Did I use an appropriate approach to synthesizing the findings from across the papers included in my review?
- Have I made the findings, and how these were reached, clear?
- Is my discussion focused on the findings from the review?
- Are my conclusions firmly based on the findings from the review?
- Do my conclusions address the review question and fulfil the study aims?
- Do my recommendations arise directly from my conclusions?
- Have I provided clear and consistent rationales for the decisions made throughout my review?

References

Allen, M., Titsworth, S. and Hunt, S.K. (2009) *Quantitative Research in Communication*. Los Angeles. Sage.

Anderson, C. (2010) Presenting and evaluating qualitative research. *American Journal of Pharmaceutical Education* 74(8) Article 141.

Astin, F. (2009) A beginner's guide to appraising a qualitative research paper. *British Journal of Cardiac Nursing* 4(11) 530–3.

Aveyard, H. (2014) *Doing a Literature Review in Health and Social Care: a practical guide (3rd edition)*. Maidenhead. Open University Press.

Balls, P. (2009) Phenomenology in nursing research: methodology, interviewing and transcribing. *Nursing Times* 105(32–3) 30–3.

Bannigan, K. and Spring, H. (2015) Doing quicker literature reviews well: the search for high-quality evidence. *International Journal of Therapy and Rehabilitation* 22(4) 158.

Barnett-Page, E. and Thomas, J. (2009) Methods for the synthesis of qualitative research: a critical review. *BMC Medical Research Methodology* 9(59) DOI: 10.1186/1471-2288-9-59.

Beauchamp, T.L. and Childress, J.F. (2013) *Principles of Biomedical Ethics (7th edition)*. Oxford. Oxford University Press.

Bettany-Saltikov, J. (2010) Learning how to undertake a systematic review: part 1. *Nursing Standard* 24(50) 47–55.

Bingham, R.J. (2014) Sharing the Wisdom of Nursing by Writing for Publication. *Nursing for Women's Health* 18(6) 523–9.

Boote, D.N. and Beile, P. (2005) Scholars before researchers. *Educational Researcher* 34(6) 3–15.

Booth, A. (2004) Formulating answerable questions, Chapter 6 pp. 59–64, in A. Booth and A. Brice (Eds) *Evidence Based Practice for Information Professionals*. London. Facet Publishing.

Booth, A. (2006) Clear and present questions: formulating questions for evidence based practice. *Library Hi Tech* 24(3) 355–68.

Booth, A. (2015) Observation, Chapter 31 pp. 426–39, in K. Gerrish and J. Lathlean (Eds) *The Research Process in Nursing (7th edition)*. Chichester. Wiley-Blackwell.

Boren, S.A. and Moxley, D. (2015) Systematically Reviewing the Literature: Building the Evidence for Health Care Quality. *Health Management and Informatics* 112(1) 58–62.

Borg Debono, V., Zhang, S., Ye, C., Paul, J., Arya, A., Hurlburt, L., Murthy, Y. and Thabane, L. (2013) A look at the potential association between PICOT framing of a research question and the quality of reporting of analgesia RCTs. *BMC Anesthesiology* 13(1) 44 doi: 10.1186/1471-2253-13-44.

Bradley, E.H., Curry, L.A. and Devers, K.J. (2007) Qualitative Data Analysis for Health Services Research: Developing Taxonomy, Themes, and Theory. *Health Services Research* 42(4) 1758–72.

Bragge, P. (2010) Asking good clinical research questions and choosing the right study design. *Injury* 41 Supplement 1 S3–S6 doi: 10.1016/j.injury.2010.04.016.

Brannan, D. (2015) The benefits of a bigger toolbox: mixed methods in psychological research. *Psi Chi Journal of Psychological Research* 20(4) 258–63.

Brazabon, T. (2007) *The University of Google.* Aldershot. Ashgate.

Brouwers, M., Kho, M.E., Browman, G.P., Cluzeau, F., Feder, G., Fervers, B., Hanna, S. and Makarski, J. on behalf of the AGREE Next Steps Consortium (2010) AGREE II: Advancing guideline development, reporting and evaluation in healthcare. *Canadian Medical Association Journal* Dec. 182: E839–42. doi: 10.1503/cmaj.090449.

Bryman, A. (2014) June 1989 and beyond: Julia Brannen's contribution to mixed methods research. *International Journal of Social Research Methodology* 17(2) 121–31.

Burls, A. (2009) *What is critical appraisal?* Available at www.whatisseries.co.uk/what-is-critical-appraisal/ (accessed 26 July 2016).

Burns, N. and Grove, S.K. (2005) *The Practice of Nursing Research: conduct, critique and utilisation (5th edition).* Philadelphia. WB Saunders.

Burns, P.B., Rohrich, R.J. and Chung, K.C. (2011) The Levels of Evidence and their role in Evidence-Based Medicine. *Plastic and Reconstructive Surgery* 128(1) 305–10.

Cameron, E. and Green, M. (2009) *Making Sense of Change Management: A Complete Guide to the Models, Tools and Techniques of Organizational Change (2nd edition).* London. Kogan Page.

Campos, C.J.G. and Turato, E.R. (2009) Content analysis in studies using the clinical-qualitative method: application and perspectives. *Revista Latino-Americana de Enfermagem* 17(2) 259–64.

Cann, A. (2011) *Social Media: a guide for researchers.* Available at www.rin.ac.uk/system/files/attachments (accessed 18 November 2016).

Carman, M.J., Wolf, L.A., Henderson, D., Kamienski, M., Koziol-McLain, J., Manton, A. and Moon, M.D. (2013) Developing your clinical question: the key to successful research. *Journal of Emergency Nursing* 39(3) 299–301.

Carter, B., Cummings, J. and Cooper, L. (2007) An exploration of best practice in multi-agency working and the experiences of families of children with complex health needs. What works well and what needs to be done to improve practice for the future? *Journal of Clinical Nursing* 16(3) 527–39. doi:10.1111/j.1365-2702.2006.01554.x.

Christenbery, T.L. and Latham, T.G. (2013) Creating effective scholarly posters: A guide for DNP students. *Journal of the American Association of Nurse Practitioners* 25(1) 16–23.

Claydon, L.S. (2015) Rigour in quantitative research. *Nursing Standard* 29(47) 43–8.

Cleary, M., Horsfall, J. and Hayter, M. (2014) Qualitative research: quality results? *Journal of Advanced Nursing* 70(4) 711–13.

Collins Dictionaries (2014) *Collins English Dictionary.* Glasgow. Collins.

Cooke, A., Smith, D. and Booth, A. (2012) Beyond PICO: The SPIDER Tool for Qualitative Evidence Synthesis. *Qualitative Health Research* 22(10) 1435–43.

Cooperrider, D.L. and Whitney, D. (1999) Appreciative inquiry: A positive revolution in change, Chapter 15 pp. 245–61, in P. Holman and T. Devane (Eds) *The Change Handbook: Group methods for shaping the future*. San Francisco. Berrett-Koehler.

Cooperrider, D.L., Whitney, D. and Stavros, J.M. (2008) *Appreciative Inquiry Handbook: For leaders of change (2nd edition)*. Brunswick, OH. Crown Custom.

da Costa Santos, C.M., de Mattos Pimenta, C.A. and Nobre, M.R.C. (2007) The PICO strategy for the research question construction and evidence search. *Revista Latino-Americana de Enfermagem* 15(3) 508–11.

Critical Appraisal Skills Programme (CASP project). Available at www.casp-uk.net/#!checklists/cb36 (accessed 27 December 2015).

Crombie, I.K. and Davies, H.T.O. (2009) *What is meta-analysis? (2nd edition)*. Available at http://vivrolfe.com/ProfDoc/Assets/Crombie%20What%20is%20a%20meta%20analysis.pdf (accessed 18 November 2016).

Cronin, P., Ryan, F. and Coughlan, M. (2008) Undertaking a literature review: a step-by-step approach. *British Journal of Nursing* 17(1) 38–43.

de la Cuesta Benjumea, C. (2015) The quality of qualitative research: from evaluation to attainment. *Texto & Contexto – Enfermagem* 24(3) 883–90.

Davey, R. (2007) Making an effective bid: developing a successful research proposal. *Clinician in Management* 15(3/4) 137–44.

Denscombe, M. (2012) *Research Proposals, a Practical Guide* ('Open Up Study Skills' series) Maidenhead. McGraw-Hill Education.

Egerod, I., Bergbom, I., Lindahl, B., Henricson, M., Granberg-Axell, A. and Storli, S. (2015) The Patient experience of intensive care: A meta-synthesis of Nordic studies. *International Journal of Nursing Studies* 52(8) 1354–61.

European Commission (2004) *Aid Delivery Methods. Volume 1: Project Cycle Management Guidelines*. Brussels. European Commission, Europaid Corporation Office.

Finchman, J.E. (2008) Response Rates and Responsiveness for Surveys, Standards, and the Journal. *American Journal of Pharmaceutical Education* 72(2) Article 43.

Freshwater, D. and Holloway, I. (2015) Narrative Research, Chapter 17, pp. 224–35, in K. Gerrish and J. Lathlean (Eds) *The Research Process in Nursing (7th edition)*. Chichester. Wiley-Blackwell.

Garavaglia, B. (2008) The problem with root cause analysis. *Nursing Homes* February 38–9.

Glasper, E.A. and Peate, I. (2013) Writing for publication. *British Journal of Nursing* 22(16) 964–8.

Glasziou, P., Vandenbroucke, J. and Chalmers, P. (2004) Assessing the quality of research. *British Medical Journal* 328(7430) 39–41.

Golder, S., Loke, Y.K. and Zorzela, L. (2014) Comparison of search strategies in systematic reviews of adverse effects to other systematic reviews. *Health Information and Libraries Journal* 31(2) 92–105.

Gopikrishna, V. (2010) A report on case reports. *Journal of Conservative Dentistry* 13(4) 265–71.

Greenhalgh, T. (2010) Statistics for the non-statistician, Chapter 5 pp. 61–76, in T. Greenhalgh *How to Read a Paper: The Basics of Evidence-Based Medicine (4th edition)*. Chichester. Wiley-Blackwell.

Guyatt, G.H., Oxman, A.D., Kunz, R., Atkins, D., Brozek, J., Vist, G., Alderson, P., Glasziou, P., Falck-Ytter, Y. and Schunemann, H.J. (2011) GRADE guidelines: 2. Framing the question and deciding on important outcomes. *Journal of Clinical Epidemiology* 64(4): 395–400.

Haidich, A.B. (2010) Meta-analysis in medical research. *Hippokratia* 14(Suppl. 1) 29–37.

Halcomb, E.J., Andrew, S. and Brannen, J. (2009) Introduction to mixed methods research for nursing and the health sciences, Chapter 1 pp. 3–12, in S. Andrews and E.J. Halcomb (Eds) *Mixed Methods Research for Nursing and the Health Sciences*. Chichester. Wiley-Blackwell.

Happell, B. (2008) Writing for publication: a practical guide. *Nursing Standard* 22(28) 35–40.

Happell, B. (2009) Presenting with precision: preparing and delivering a polished conference presentation. *Nurse Researcher* 16(3) 45–56.

Hasson, F., McKenna, H. and Keeney, S. (2015) Surveys, Chapter 19 pp. 254–65, in K. Gerrish and J. Lathlean (Eds) *The Research Process in Nursing (7th edition)*. Chichester. Wiley-Blackwell.

Heale, R. and Twycross, A. (2015) Validity and reliability in quantitative studies. *Evidence Based Nursing* 18(3) 66–7.

Hebda, T. and Czar, P. (2009) *Handbook of Informatics for Nurses and Healthcare Professionals (4th edition)*. Upper Saddle River, NJ. Pearson Education Inc.

Hemingway, P. and Brereton, N. (2009) *What is a systematic review? (2nd edition)*. Available at http://docplayer.net/84335-What-is-a-systematic-review.html (accessed 18 November 2016).

Hess, G.R., Tosney, K.W. and Liegel, L.H. (2009) Creating effective poster presentations: AMEE Guide no. 40. *Medical Teacher* 31(4) 319–21.

Higgins, J.P.T. and Green, S. (2011) *Cochrane Handbook for Systematic Reviews of Interventions* Version 5.1.0 [updated March 2011]. The Cochrane Collaboration. Available from http://handbook.cochrane.org (accessed 26 July 2016).

Hill, T. and Lewicki, P. (2007) *Statistics Methods and Applications*. Tulsa, OK. Statsoft.

Hoe, J. and Hoare, Z. (2012) Understanding quantitative research: part 1. *Nursing Standard* 27(15–17) 52–7.

Holland, M. (2007) *Advanced Searching: Researcher Guide*. Bournemouth. Bournemouth University.

Holloway, I. and Galvin, K.T. (2015) Grounded Theory, Chapter 14 pp. 184–97, in K. Gerrish and J. Lathlean (Eds) *The Research Process in Nursing (7th edition)*. Chichester. Wiley-Blackwell.

Houghton, C., Casey, D., Shaw, D. and Murphy, K. (2013) Rigour in qualitative case-study research. *Nurse Researcher* 20(4)12–17.

Hovland, I. (2005) *Successful Communication: A Toolkit for Researchers and Civil Society Organisations*. London. Overseas Development Institute. Available at www.odi.org.uk/resources/docs/192.pdf (accessed 23 July 2016).

Hunt, K. and Lathlean, J. (2015) Sampling, Chapter 13 pp. 172–83, in K. Gerrish and J. Lathlean (Eds) *The Research Process in Nursing (7th edition)*. Chichester. Wiley-Blackwell.

Hunter, J.P., Saratzis, A., Sutton, J.A., Boucher, R.H., Sayers, R.D. and Bown, M.J. (2014) Meta-analyses of proportion studies, funnel plots were found to be an inaccurate method of assessing publication bias. *Journal of Clinical Epidemiology* 67(8) 897–903.

Iles, V. and Cranfield, S. (2004) *Managing Change in the NHS. Developing Change Management Skills: A resource for health care professionals and managers*. London. National Co-ordinating Centre for NHS Service Delivery and Organization Research and Development.

Jack, L.J., Hayes, S.C., Scharalda, J.G., Stetson, B., Jones-Jack, N.H., Valliere, M., Kirchain, W.R., Fagen, M. and LeBlanc, C. (2010) Appraising Quantitative Research in Health Education: Guidelines for Public Health Educators. *Health Promotion Practice* 11(2)161–5.

Jones, M. and Rattray, J. (2015) Questionnaire design, Chapter 30 pp. 412–25, in K. Gerrish and J. Lathlean (Eds) *The Research Process in Nursing (7th edition)*. Chichester. Wiley-Blackwell.

Jootun, D. and McGhee, G. (2009) Reflexivity: promoting rigour in qualitative research. *Nursing Standard* 23(2) 42–6.

Kamienski, M., Carman, M.J., Wolf, L.A., Henderson, D. and Manton, A. (2013) Searching the literature: what is known (and not known) about your topic? *Journal of Emergency Nursing* 39(4) 395–7.

Keating, S. and Tocco, S. (2013) Getting to the root of the root-cause analysis problem. *American Nurse Today* 8(8) 56–9.

Kohfeldt, D. and Langhaut, R.D. (2012) The Five Whys Method: A Tool for Developing Problem Definitions in Collaboration with Children. *Journal of Community and Applied Social Psychology* 22(4) 316–29.

Koster, R.L.P. and Lemelin, R.H. (2009) Appreciative inquiry in rural tourism: A case study from Canada. *Tourism Geographies* 11(2) 256–69.

Kumar, R. (2005) *Research methodology: a step-by-step guide for beginners*. London. Sage.

Kung, S., Giles, D. and Hagan, B. (2013) Applying an Appreciative Inquiry Process to a Course Evaluation in Higher Education. *International Journal of Teaching and Learning in Higher Education* 25(1) 29–37.

Latino, R.J. (2004) Optimizing FMEA and RCA efforts in health care. *Journal of Healthcare Risk Management* 24(3) 21–8.

Le Boiutelier, C., Chevalier, A., Lawrence, V., Leamy, M., Bird, V.J., Macpherson, R., Williams, J. and Slade, M. (2015) Staff understanding of recovery-orientated mental health practice: a systematic review and narrative synthesis. *Implementation Science* 10(87) DOI: 10.1186/s13012-015-0275-4.

Levy, Y. and Ellis, T.J. (2006) A Systems Approach to Conduct an Effective Literature Review in Support of Information Systems Research. *Informing Science Journal* 9 181–212.

Lincoln, Y.S. and Guba, E.G. (1985) *Naturalistic Inquiry*. Newbury Park, CA. Sage Publications.

Lipowski, E.E. (2008) Developing great research questions. *American Journal of Health Systems Pharmacy* 65(17) 1667–70.

Lunenburg, F.C. and Irby, B.J. (2008) *Writing a Successful Thesis or Dissertation: Tips and Strategies for Students in the Social and Behavioral Sciences.* Thousand Oaks, CA. Corwin Press.

McGeehan, B., Debbage, S., Gilsenan, I., Jennings, A., Jennings, C., Laker, S., Thompson, S. and Beastall, H. (2009) Supporting clinical innovation: An organization-wide approach to practice-based development. *Practice Development in Health Care* 8(1) 18–27.

MacInnes, J. (2009) Mixed methods studies: a guide to critical appraisal. *British Journal of Cardiac Nursing* 4(12) 588–91.

Malicki, M. and Marusic, A. on behalf of the OPEN (2014) Is there a solution to publication bias? Researchers call for changes in dissemination of clinical research results. *Journal of Clinical Epidemiology* 67(10) 1103–10.

Maltby, J., Williams, G.A., McGarry, J. and Day, L. (2010) *Research Methods for Nursing and Healthcare.* Harlow. Pearson Education.

Martin, W.E. and Bridgmon, K.D. (2012) *Quantitative and statistical research methods: from hypothesis to results for all of them.* San Francisco. Jossey-Bass.

Methley, A.M., Campbell, S., Chew-Graham, C., McNally, R. and Cheraghi-Sohi, S. (2014) PICO, PICOS and SPIDER: a comparison study of specificity and sensitivity in three search tools for qualitative systematic reviews. *BMC Health Services Research* 14(1) 579 DOI: 10.1186/s12913-014-0579-0.

Moon, M.D., Baker, K., Carman, M.J., Clark, P.R., Henderson, D., Manton, A. and Zavotsky, K.E. (2013) Evaluating qualitative research studies for use in the clinical setting. *Journal of Emergency Nursing* 39(5) 508–10.

Moore, M. (2008) Appreciative inquiry: The why? The what? The how? *Practice Development in Health Care* 7(4) 214–20.

Moreno, S.G., Sutton, A.J., Turner, E.H., Abrams, K.R., Cooper, N.J., Palmer, T.M. and Ades, A.E. (2009) Novel methods to deal with publication biases: secondary analysis of antidepressant trials in the FDA trial registry database and related journal publications. *British Medical Journal* 339(7719) 493–8.

Morse, J.M. (2012) *Qualitative Health Research: Creating a New Discipline.* Walnut Creek, CA. Left Coast Press.

Murphy, S.L., Robinson, J.C. and Lin, S.H. (2009) Conducting Systematic reviews to inform occupational therapy practice. *The American Journal of Occupational Therapy* 68(3) 363–8.

Murray, R. (2011) *How to Write a Thesis.* Maidenhead. Open University Press.

National Health Service Health Research Authority (2009) *Defining Research.* London. Health Research Authority. Available from www.hra.nhs.uk/resources/before-you-apply/is-it-research/ (accessed 26 July 2016).

National Institute for Health and Care Excellence (2014) *Developing NICE Guidelines: The Manual.* London. NICE.

Naude, L., van den Bergh, T.J. and Kruger, I.S. (2014) Learning to like learning: an appreciative inquiry into emotions in education. *Social Psychology of Education* 17(2) 211–28.

Nayak, B.K. and Hazra, A.I. (2011) How to choose the right statistical test? *Indian Journal of Ophthalmology* 59(2) 85–6.

Nelson, A.E., Dumville, J. and Torgerson, D. (2015) Experimental Research, Chapter 18 pp. 236–53, in K. Gerrish and J. Lathlean (Eds) *The Research Process in Nursing (7th edition)*. Chichester. Wiley-Blackwell.

Offredy, M. and Vickers, P.S. (2010) *Developing a Healthcare Research Proposal: An Interactive Student Guide*. Chichester. Wiley-Blackwell.

Okes, D. (2008) The Human Side of Root Cause Analysis. *Journal for Quality and Participation* 31(3) 20–9.

Onitilo, A.A. (2014) Is It Time for the Cochrane Collaboration to Reconsider Its Meta-Analysis Methodology? *Clinical Medicine and Research* 12(1–2) 2–3.

Parahoo, K. (2014) *Nursing Research: Principles, Process and Issues (3rd edition)*. Basingstoke. Palgrave Macmillan.

Parish, C. (2012) Creating the right conditions for person-centred care to flourish. *Learning Disability Practice* 15(9) 6–8.

Parkin, P. (2009) *Managing Change in Healthcare Using Action Research*. London. Sage.

Paton, R.A. and McCalman, J. (2008) *Change Management: a guide to effective implementation (3rd edition)*. London. Sage.

Pereira, H. (2012) Rigour in phenomenological research: reflections of a novice nurse researcher. *Nurse Researcher* 19(3) 16–19.

Pilnick, A. and Swift, J.A. (2010) Qualitative research in nutrition and dietetics: assessing quality. *Journal of Human Nutrition and Dietetics* 24(3) 209–14.

Polit, D.F. and Beck, C.T. (2006) *Essentials of Nursing Research: Methods, Appraisal and Utilisation (6th edition)*. Philadelphia. Lippincott Williams and Wilkins.

Poojary, S.A. and Bagadia, J.D. (2014) Reviewing literature for research: Doing it the right way. *Indian Journal of Sexually Transmitted Diseases and AIDS* 35(2) 85–91.

Quick, J. and Hall, S. (2015) Part one: An introduction to the research process. *Journal of Perioperative Practice* 25(4) 78–82.

Randall, R. (2011) Ask 'Why?' five times to dig up the real root cause of a problem. *Central Penn Business Journal* 1 July.

Reed, J. (2007) *Appreciative Inquiry: Research for change*. Thousand Oaks, CA. Sage.

Ren, D. (2009) Understanding statistical hypothesis testing. *Journal of Emergency Nursing* 35(1) 57–9.

Riva, J.J., Malik, K.M.P., Burnie, S.J., Endicott, A.R. and Busse, J.W. (2012) What is your research question? An introduction to the PICOT format for clinicians. *Journal of the Canadian Chiropractor's Association* 56(3) 167–71.

Roberts, P. and Priest, H. (2006) Reliability and validity in research. *Nursing Standard* 20(44) 41–5.

Roberts, S.H. and Bailey, J.E. (2011) Incentives and barriers to lifestyle interventions for people with severe mental illness: a narrative synthesis of quantitative, qualitative and mixed methods studies. *Journal of Advanced Nursing* 67(4) 690–708.

Rodgers, M., Sowden, A., Petticrew, M., Arai, L., Roberts, H., Britten, N. and Poppay, J. (2009) Testing Methodological Guidance on the Conduct of Narrative Synthesis in Systematic Reviews: Effectiveness of Interventions to Promote Smoke Alarm Ownership and Function. *Evaluation* 15(1) 49–74.

Roecker, C. (2012) Hierarchy of evidence awareness saves time. *Journal of the American Chiropractic Association* March–April 7–10.

Ross, T. (2012) *A Survival Guide For Health Research Methods*. Maidenhead. McGraw-Hill Education.

Rowlands, I., Nicholas, D., Russell, B., Canty, N. and Watkinson, A. (2011) Social media use in the research workflow. *Learned Publishing* 24(3) 183–95.

Ryan, F., Coughlan, M. and Cronin, P. (2007) Step-by-step guide to critiquing research. Part 2: qualitative research. *British Journal of Nursing* 16(12) 738–44.

Ryan, R. (2013) *Cochrane Consumers and Communication Review Group: data synthesis and analysis*. Available at http://cccrg.cochrane.org (accessed 17 May 2016).

Saba, V.K. and McCormick, K.A. (2001) *Essentials of Computers for Nurses (3rd edition)*. New York. McGraw-Hill.

Saini, M. and Shlonsky, A. (2012) *Systematic synthesis of qualitative research. Pocket Guides to Social Research Methods*. New York. Oxford University Press.

Siddiqi, N. (2011) Publication bias in epidemiological studies. *Central European Journal of Public Health* 19(2) 118–20.

Snilstveit, B., Oliver, S. and Vojtkova, M. (2012) Narrative approaches to systematic review and synthesis of evidence for international development policy and practice. *Journal of Development Effectiveness* 4(3) 409–29.

Thames Valley Literature Review Standards Group (2006) *The Literature Searching Process: protocol for researchers*. London. Thames Valley Health Libraries Network.

Thomas, E. (2005) An introduction to medical statistics for health care professionals: Hypothesis tests and estimation. *Musculoskeletal Care* 3(2)102–8.

Tod, A. (2015) Interviewing, Chapter 28 pp. 386–99, in K. Gerrish and J. Lathlean (Eds) *The Research Process in Nursing (7th edition)*. Chichester. Wiley-Blackwell.

Todres, L. (2005) Clarifying the life-world: descriptive phenomenology, Chapter 7 pp. 104–24, in I. Holloway (Ed.) *Qualitative Research in Healthcare*. Maidenhead. Open University Press.

Tolmie, A., McAteer, E. and Muijs, D. (2011) *Quantitative Methods in Educational and Social Research Using SPSS*. Maidenhead. Open University Press.

Tungpunkom, P. and Turale, S. (2014) Considering knowledge and reviewing literature: the case of systematic reviews. *Pacific Rim International Journal of Nursing Research* 18(4) 271–3.

Turnbull, J. and Lathlean, J. (2015) Mixed methods research, Chapter 27 pp. 371–83, in K. Gerrish and J. Lathlean (Eds) *The Research Process in Nursing (7th edition)*. Chichester. Wiley-Blackwell.

Uman, L.S. (2011) Systematic Reviews and Meta-Analyses. *Journal of the Canadian Academy of Child and Adolescent Psychiatry* 20(1) 57–9.

Venkatesh, V., Brown, S.A. and Bala, H. (2013) Bridging the qualitative-quantitative divide: guidelines for conducting mixed methods research in information systems. *MIS Quarterly* 37(1) 21–54.

Walsh, K., Jordan, Z. and Appolloni, L. (2009) The problematic art of conversation: communication and health practice evolution. *Practice Development in Health Care* 8(3) 166–79.

Waltho, D., Kaur, M.N., Haynes, R.B., Farrokhyar, F. and Thoma, A. (2015) Users' guide to the surgical literature: how to perform a high-quality literature search. *Canadian Journal of Surgery* 58(5) 349–58.

White, B. (2011) *Mapping Your Thesis: The Comprehensive Manual of Theory and Techniques for Masters and Doctoral Research*. Melbourne. ACER.

Whiting, L.S. (2008) Semi-structured interviews: guidance for novice researchers. *Nursing Standard* 22(23) 35–40.

Willig, C. (2008) *Introducing qualitative research in psychology. Adventures in theory and method* (2nd edition). Maidenhead. Open University Press.

Wilson, M. and Gochyyev, P. (2013) Psychometrics, Chapter 1 pp. 3–30, in T. Teo (Ed.) *Handbook of Quantitative Methods for Educational Research*. Rotterdam. Sense Publishers.

Windish, D.M. and Diener-West, M. (2006) A Clinician-educator's roadmap to choosing and interpreting statistical tests. *Journal of General Internal Medicine* 21(6) 656–60.

Yazdani, A.A. and Tavakkoli-Moghaddam, R. (2012) Integration of the fish bone diagram, brainstorming, and AHP method for problem solving and decision making – a case study. *International Journal of Advanced Manufacturing Technology* 63 651–7.

Zitomer, M.R. and Goodwin, D. (2014) Gauging the Quality of Qualitative Research in Adapted Physical Activity. *Adapted Physical Activity Quarterly* 31(3) 193–218.

Index

Page numbers in *italics* denote tables, those in **bold** denote figures.